Mechanical Ventilation

Pittsburgh Critical Care Medicine Series

Published and Forthcoming Titles
in the Pittsburgh Critical Care Medicine Series

Mechanical Ventilation

Physiology and Practice

Second Edition

John W. Kreit, MD
Professor of Medicine and Anesthesiology
Division of Pulmonary, Allergy, and Critical Care Medicine
University of Pittsburgh School of Medicine
Pittsburgh, PA

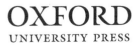

OXFORD
UNIVERSITY PRESS

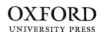

Oxford University Press is a department of the University of Oxford. It furthers
the University's objective of excellence in research, scholarship, and education
by publishing worldwide. Oxford is a registered trade mark of Oxford University
Press in the UK and certain other countries.

Published in the United States of America by Oxford University Press
198 Madison Avenue, New York, NY 10016, United States of America.

© Oxford University Press 2018

Library of Congress Cataloging-in-Publication Data
Names: Kreit, John W., author.
Title: Mechanical ventilation : physiology and practice / by John W. Kreit.
Description: Second edition. | Oxford ; New York : Oxford University Press, [2018] |
Preceded by Mechanical ventilation / edited by John W. Kreit. c2013.
Identifiers: LCCN 2017022820 | ISBN 9780190670085 (pbk. : alk. paper)
Subjects: | MESH: Respiration, Artificial | Ventilators, Mechanical
Classification: LCC RC735.I5 | NLM WF 145 | DDC 615.8/3620284—dc23
LC record available at https://lccn.loc.gov/2017022820

This material is not intended to be, and should not be considered, a substitute for medical
or other professional advice. Treatment for the conditions described in this material is highly
dependent on the individual circumstances. And, while this material is designed to offer
accurate information with respect to the subject matter covered and to be current as of the
time it was written, research and knowledge about medical and health issues is constantly
evolving and dose schedules for medications are being revised continually, with new side
effects recognized and accounted for regularly. Readers must therefore always check the
product information and clinical procedures with the most up-to-date published product
information and data sheets provided by the manufacturers and the most recent codes
of conduct and safety regulation. The publisher and the authors make no representations
or warranties to readers, express or implied, as to the accuracy or completeness of
this material. Without limiting the foregoing, the publisher and the authors make no
representations or warranties as to the accuracy or efficacy of the drug dosages mentioned
in the material. The authors and the publisher do not accept, and expressly disclaim, any
responsibility for any liability, loss or risk that may be claimed or incurred as a consequence
of the use and/or application of any of the contents of this material.

9 8 7 6 5 4 3 2 1

Printed by Webcom Inc., Canada

To my wife, Marilyn, and my children, Jennifer and Brian, for their love and support

To Ellison, Bennett, Cora, and Avery, who have brought joy to my life

To my fellows—past, present, and future

Contents

Preface

Mechanical ventilation is an essential, life-sustaining therapy for many critically ill patients. As technology has evolved, clinicians have been presented with an increasing number of ventilator options as well as an ever-expanding and confusing list of terms, abbreviations, and acronyms. Unfortunately, this has made it extremely difficult for students and physicians at all levels of training to truly understand mechanical ventilation and to optimally manage patients with respiratory failure. This volume of the Pittsburgh Critical Care Medicine Series was written to address this problem. This handbook provides students, residents, fellows, and practicing physicians with a clear explanation of essential pulmonary and cardiovascular physiology, terms and acronyms, and ventilator modes and breath types. It describes how mechanical ventilators work and explains clearly and concisely how to write ventilator orders, how to manage patients with many different causes of respiratory failure, how to "wean" patients from the ventilator, and much more. *Mechanical Ventilation* is meant to be carried and used at the bedside and to allow everyone who cares for critically ill patients to master this essential therapy.

Mechanical Ventilation

Section 1

Essential Physiology

Despite its enticing title, I know that you're probably thinking about skipping this section and diving right into the second or third part of this book. That would be a mistake. I'm not saying this just because I'm the author and because my feelings are easily hurt. I'm saying it because I know that you want an in-depth understanding of mechanical ventilation, and that requires a working knowledge of certain essential aspects of pulmonary and cardiovascular physiology. Sure, you can learn a lot by reading later chapters in this book, but to really master the subject, you have to start at the beginning. You have to start with the first three chapters, which provide the foundation for all the chapters that follow.

I know that physiology is usually presented in a rather complex and dry format, and that's a shame, because it keeps people from seeing how important it really is. I will do everything I can to make this material interesting, straightforward, and relevant. So let's get started!

Chapter 1

Respiratory Mechanics

The *respiratory system* consists of the lungs and the chest wall. The chest wall includes the rib cage and all the tissues and muscles attached to it, including the diaphragm. The function of the respiratory system is to remove carbon dioxide (CO_2) from, and add oxygen (O_2) to, the mixed venous blood that is pumped through the pulmonary circulation by the right ventricle. To do this, two interrelated processes must occur:

- *Ventilation*—the repetitive bulk movement of gas into and out of the lungs
- *Gas exchange*—several processes that together allow the respiratory system to maintain a normal arterial partial pressure of O_2 and CO_2

Ventilation can occur only when the respiratory system expands above and then returns to its resting or equilibrium volume. This is just a fancy way of saying that ventilation depends on our ability to breathe. Although for most people, breathing requires very little effort and even less thought, it's nevertheless a fairly complex process. In fact, ventilation can occur only when sufficient pressure is applied to overcome two forces that oppose the movement of the respiratory system. The interaction of these *applied* and *opposing* forces is referred to as the "mechanics of ventilation," or *respiratory mechanics*.

Opposing Forces

Elastic Recoil

If you were to watch lung transplant surgery or an autopsy, you would see that the lungs deflate when they're taken out of the thoracic cavity. If you looked closely, you would also notice that the chest wall increases in volume once the lungs are removed. This occurs because the isolated lungs and chest wall each have their own resting or *equilibrium volumes*. As you can see from Figure 1.1, any change from these volumes requires an increasing amount of applied pressure. So, if you think about it, the lungs and the chest wall act just like metal springs. The more they're stretched or compressed, the greater the amount of pressure needed to overcome their inherent *elastic recoil*.

The elastic recoil of the lungs and chest wall has two sources:

- *Tissue forces* result from the stretching of so-called elastic elements—elastin and collagen in the lungs, and cartilage, bone, and muscle in the chest wall.

- *Surface forces* are unique to the lungs and result from the surface tension generated by the layer of surfactant that coats the inside of each alveolus.

Pressure–Volume Relationships

The elastic recoil of the lungs, chest wall, and intact respiratory system is commonly depicted by graphs that show the pressure needed to maintain a specific volume. To help you understand these *volume–pressure curves*, I first want to spend some time looking at the properties of the lung spring and the chest wall spring shown in Figure 1.1. The relationship between the length of each "spring" and the pressure needed to balance its elastic recoil (also known as the *elastic recoil pressure*) is shown in Figure 1.2. As you can see, as the lung

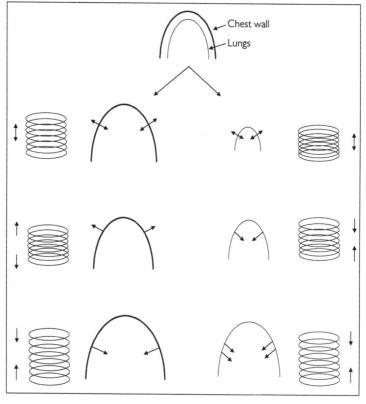

Figure 1.1 When separated from each other, the lungs recoil inward and the chest wall expands outward to reach their individual equilibrium volumes (*double-sided arrows*). Any change from these volumes requires an increasing amount of applied pressure to balance increasing inward or outward elastic recoil (*arrows*). In this way, the lungs and chest wall act just like metal springs.

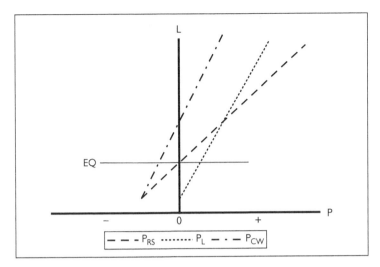

Figure 1.2 Relationship between pressure (P) and length (L) of the lung spring (P_L), the chest wall spring (P_{CW}), and the "respiratory system" (P_{RS}). Note that, at any length, P_{RS} is the sum of P_L and P_{CW}. The resting or equilibrium length is the point at which each line crosses the Y-axis and $P = 0$. Increasing outward (+) or inward (−) pressure is required to balance elastic recoil as the chest wall spring and the "respiratory system" are stretched above or compressed below their equilibrium lengths. The "respiratory system" reaches its equilibrium (EQ) length when the inward recoil of the lung spring is exactly balanced by the outward recoil of the chest wall spring.

spring is stretched, more and more applied pressure (P_L) is needed. Similarly, increasing outward or inward pressure (P_{CW}) is needed to lengthen or shorten the chest wall spring. Notice that the resting or equilibrium length of each spring is the point at which it crosses the Y-axis and applied pressure (and elastic recoil) is zero.

Now let's see what happens when we hook these two springs together in parallel (side by side). After all, the real lungs and chest wall are attached by a very thin layer of pleural fluid and function together as a single unit. Figure 1.2 shows that the elastic properties of this "respiratory system" are determined by the sum of its two individual pressure–length curves. In other words, at any length, the pressure needed to balance the elastic recoil of the "respiratory system" (P_{RS}) is the sum of P_L and P_{CW}. Notice that the resting length of the "respiratory system" is the point at which the inward recoil of the lung spring is exactly balanced by the outward recoil of the chest wall spring and P_{RS} is zero.

How can this possibly be relevant to pulmonary physiology? It turns out that the *length–pressure* curves of our springs are remarkably similar to the *volume–pressure* curves of the lungs, chest wall, and respiratory system. So if you understand the concepts shown in Figure 1.2, you're well on your way to understanding everything you need to know about the elastic properties of the respiratory system.

Skeptical? Take a look at Figure 1.3, which shows the elastic recoil pressure of the respiratory system and its components at every volume between total lung capacity (TLC) and residual volume (RV). These curves are generated by having a subject relax his or her respiratory muscles at a number of different volumes while a shutter attached to a mouthpiece prevents exhalation.

At each volume, the pressure in the pleural space (P_{PL}) and the airway (P_{AW}) just proximal to the shutter are measured, and the *transmural* pressure (the internal or *intramural* pressure minus the external or *extramural* pressure) of the lungs ($P_{L_{TM}}$), chest wall (Pcw_{TM}), and respiratory system ($P_{RS_{TM}}$) are calculated (Figure 1.4).

Note that: (1) in the absence of air flow, P_{AW} and alveolar pressure (P_{ALV}) are equal; (2) P_{PL} is estimated by measuring the pressure in the esophagus (P_{ES}) with a thin, balloon-tipped catheter; and (3) pressure at the body surface (P_{BS}) is normally atmospheric pressure (P_{ATM}), which is assigned a value of zero. It's important to understand that these measurements must be performed under static (no-flow) conditions if they are to reflect only the pressure needed to overcome elastic recoil—but more about that later.

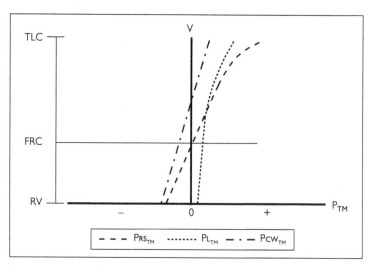

Figure 1.3 Relationship between transmural pressure (P_{TM}) and volume (V) of the lungs ($P_{L_{TM}}$), chest wall (Pcw_{TM}), and respiratory system ($P_{RS_{TM}}$). Each curve shows how much outward (+) or inward () pressure is needed to balance elastic recoil at volumes between residual volume (RV) and total lung capacity (TLC). At any volume, $P_{RS_{TM}}$ is the sum of $P_{L_{TM}}$ and Pcw_{TM}. The resting or equilibrium volume is the point at which each line crosses the Y-axis and $P_{TM} = 0$. The respiratory system reaches its equilibrium volume at functional residual capacity (FRC) when the inward recoil of the lungs is exactly balanced by the outward recoil of the chest wall.

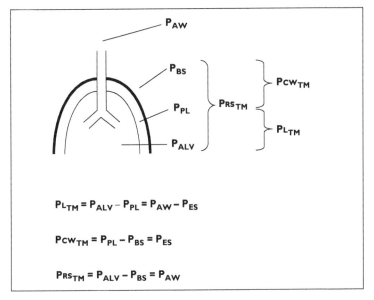

$$P_{L_{TM}} = P_{ALV} - P_{PL} = P_{AW} - P_{ES}$$

$$P_{CW_{TM}} = P_{PL} - P_{BS} = P_{ES}$$

$$P_{RS_{TM}} = P_{ALV} - P_{BS} = P_{AW}$$

Figure 1.4 The transmural pressure of the lungs ($P_{L_{TM}}$), chest wall ($P_{CW_{TM}}$), and respiratory system ($P_{RS_{TM}}$) is calculated by subtracting the pressure "outside" from the pressure "inside" each structure. Pressure at the body surface (P_{BS}) is equal to atmospheric pressure and assigned a value of zero. Pleural pressure (P_{PL}) is estimated by measuring the pressure in the lower esophagus (P_{ES}). When there is no air flow, alveolar pressure (P_{ALV}) and airway pressure (P_{AW}) are equal.

Look how much you already know about the elastic properties of the respiratory system. Just like in our spring model, the pressure needed to maintain the respiratory system at any volume is the sum of the elastic recoil pressures of the lungs and chest wall. The volume reached at the end of a relaxed or passive expiration (functional residual capacity; FRC) is the point at which the inward recoil of the lungs is exactly balanced by the outward recoil of the chest wall ($P_{RS_{TM}} = 0$). Until it reaches its equilibrium volume ($P_{CW_{TM}} = 0$), the outward recoil of the chest wall actually assists with lung inflation. At higher volumes, sufficient pressure must be applied to overcome the inward recoil of both the lungs and the chest wall. Below FRC, pressure must be applied to balance the increasing outward recoil of the chest wall.

Viscous Forces

A spring is a great metaphor for elastic recoil, because it's easy to understand that a certain amount of pressure is needed to keep it at a specific length. When we breathe, though, we have to do more than just overcome the elastic recoil of the respiratory system. We also have to drive gas into and out of the lungs through the tracheobronchial tree. This requires additional pressure

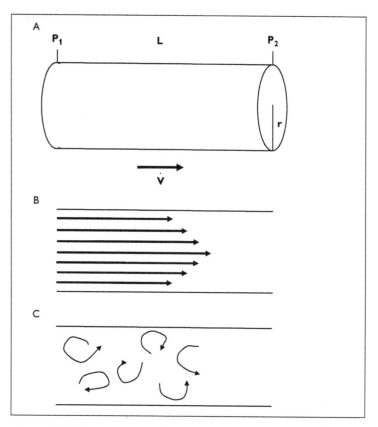

Figure 1.5 (A) The pressure gradient between the ends of a tube $(P_1 - P_2)$ is determined by the rate of gas flow $(\dot{V})$ and the radius (r) and length (L) of the tube.

(B) During laminar flow, gas moves in concentric sheets, and velocity increases toward the center of the airway.

(C) Chaotic or turbulent flow requires a much higher pressure gradient.

to overcome both the friction generated by gas molecules as they move over the surface of the airways, and the cohesive forces between these molecules. Together, these are referred to as *viscous forces*.

Pressure–Flow Relationships

The best way to understand viscous forces is to think about blowing (or sucking) air through a tube (Figure 1.5A). Air will flow through the tube only if there's a difference in *intramural* pressure (ΔP_{IM}) between its two ends. Just how much of a pressure gradient is needed depends on several factors, which are shown in this simplification of Poiseuille's equation:

$$\Delta P_{IM} \, \alpha \, \dot{V}L/r^4 \tag{1.1}$$

Here, $\dot{V}$ is the flow rate, and L is the length and r the radius of the tube. Don't worry about memorizing this equation, because, believe it or not, you already know what it says. Think about it. It simply says that you have to blow or suck harder if you want to generate a high flow rate or if the tube is either very long or very narrow. The only thing you really need to remember is that radius is the most important determinant of the pressure gradient. It's a lot harder to blow through a coffee stirrer than through a drinking straw!

Of course, the tracheobronchial tree is much more complex than a simple tube. The good news is that flow into and out of the lungs is governed by exactly the same principles. It's important to recognize, though, that Equation 1.1 is true only when flow is *laminar*—that is, when gas moves in orderly, concentric sheets (Figure 1.5B). If flow is chaotic or *turbulent* (Figure 1.5C), ΔP_{IM} varies directly with $\dot{V}^2$ and inversely with the 5th power of the airway radius. High flow, high gas density, and branching of the airways predispose to turbulent flow.

Compliance and Resistance

Elastic recoil and viscous forces play a very important role in the mechanics of ventilation, so it's helpful to be able to quantify them. Elastic recoil is most often expressed in terms of *compliance* (C), which is the ratio of the volume change (ΔV) produced by a change in *transmural* pressure (ΔP_{TM}).

$$C = \Delta V / \Delta P_{TM} \tag{1.2}$$

Notice that compliance and elastic recoil are inversely related. When elastic recoil is high, a given pressure change produces a relatively small change in volume, and compliance is low. When elastic recoil is low, the same pressure change produces a much greater change in volume, and compliance is high. By definition, compliance is a *static* measurement. In other words, it can only be calculated in the absence of flow. Since compliance is the ratio of volume and transmural pressure, it is equal to the slope of the volume–pressure curves in Figure 1.3. Notice that respiratory system compliance is highest in the tidal volume range and decreases at higher volumes.

Viscous forces are quantified by *resistance* (R), which is the ratio of the *intramural* pressure gradient (ΔP_{IM}) and the resulting flow ($\dot{V}$).

$$R = \Delta P_{IM} / \dot{V} \tag{1.3}$$

When resistance is low, a small pressure gradient is needed to generate flow. When resistance is high, a larger pressure gradient is needed. Note that resistance is a *dynamic* measurement because it can only be calculated in the presence of flow.

Although it's probably clear, I want to emphasize that ΔP is not the same in Equations 1.2 and 1.3. When used to calculate compliance, ΔP is the change in *transmural* pressure needed to balance elastic recoil. When calculating resistance, ΔP is the *intramural* pressure gradient needed to overcome viscous forces. The methods used to calculate the compliance and resistance of the respiratory system are discussed in Chapter 9.

Applied Forces

At any time during inspiration and expiration, sufficient pressure must be applied (P_{APP}) to overcome the viscous forces (P_V) and elastic recoil (P_{ER}) of the lungs and chest wall.

$$P_{APP} = P_V + P_{ER} \qquad (1.4)$$

Based on our previous discussion, P_{ER} is the transmural pressure of the respiratory system *in the absence of gas flow,* while P_V is the intramural pressure gradient driving flow. Equation 1.2 tells us that P_{ER} is equal to the change in volume (ΔV) divided by respiratory system compliance (C_{RS}), and from Equation 1.3, we know that P_V equals the product of resistance (R) and flow ($\dot{V}$). So, we can rewrite Equation 1.4 as:

$$P_{APP} = (R \times \dot{V}) + (\Delta V / C_{RS}) \qquad (1.5)$$

This is called the *equation of motion* of the respiratory system. It tells us that at any time during the respiratory cycle, the applied pressure must vary directly with resistance, flow rate, and volume and inversely with respiratory system compliance.

The pressure required during inspiration is normally supplied by the diaphragm and the other inspiratory muscles. When they are unable to perform this function, pressure must be provided by a mechanical ventilator. Let's look at how applied and opposing forces interact during both normal or *spontaneous* breathing and mechanical ventilation.

Spontaneous Ventilation

Inspiration

Figure 1.6 shows how P_{PL}, P_{ALV}, flow, and volume change throughout inspiration. Remember that the inspiratory muscles don't inflate the lungs directly. Rather, they expand the chest wall, and lung volume increases because the visceral and parietal pleura are attached by a thin layer of pleural fluid. Pleural pressure

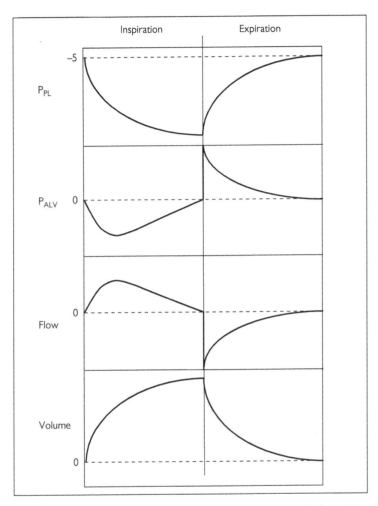

Figure 1.6 The change in pleural (P_{PL}) and alveolar (P_{ALV}) pressure, flow, and volume during a spontaneous breath. Pressure at the mouth (P_{AW}) remains zero (atmospheric pressure) during spontaneous ventilation.

is normally negative (sub-atmospheric) at end-expiration. That's because the opposing elastic recoil of the lungs and chest wall pulls the visceral and parietal pleura in opposite directions, which slightly increases the volume of the pleural space and decreases its pressure. As the inspiratory muscles expand the chest wall, lung volume and lung elastic recoil increase. This causes a further drop in P_{PL}, which reaches its lowest (most negative) value at the end of inspiration.

At end-expiration, the respiratory system is normally at its equilibrium volume, and both P_{ALV} and P_{AW} are zero (atmospheric pressure). As the inspiratory muscles expand the chest wall, the volume of the lungs increases faster than they can fill with air, and P_{ALV} falls. Since P_{AW} remains zero, this produces a pressure gradient that overcomes viscous forces and drives air into the lungs. As the lungs fill with air, P_{ALV} rises until both it and air flow return to zero at the end of inspiration. Since flow is zero at end-expiration and end-inspiration, the tidal volume during a spontaneous breath (V_T) depends only on the change in respiratory system transmural pressure and respiratory system compliance, as shown in this modification of Equation 1.2:

$$V_T = C_{RS} \times \Delta P_{RS_{TM}} \tag{1.6}$$

Watch out! Make sure you don't get confused by the differences in the pressures shown in Figures 1.3 and 1.6. Specifically, in Figure 1.3, P_{ALV} ($P_{RS_{TM}}$) and P_{PL} ($P_{CW_{TM}}$) increase with lung volume, and P_{ALV} is always equal to P_{AW}. In Figure 1.6, both P_{ALV} and P_{PL} fall, and P_{ALV} and P_{AW} are the same only at end-expiration and end-inspiration. These differences are due solely to the conditions under which the pressures are measured. Remember that the curves in Figure 1.3 are generated by having a subject relax his or her respiratory muscles at different lung volumes while a shutter prevents air from entering or leaving the lungs. The curves shown in Figure 1.6 represent "real-time" pressures during spontaneous breathing.

Since the respiratory muscles generate all the pressure (P_{MUS}) required during inspiration, the equation of motion during spontaneous ventilation can be written as:

$$P_{MUS} = (R \times \dot{V}) + \left(\Delta V / C_{RS}\right) \tag{1.7}$$

Expiration

As gas leaves the lungs and the respiratory system returns toward its equilibrium volume, pressure is required only to overcome the viscous forces produced by air flow. In the absence of expiratory muscle activity, this pressure is provided solely by the stored elastic recoil of the respiratory system. Now lung volume falls faster than air can leave, and P_{ALV} rises above P_{AW} (Figure 1.6). During such a *passive* exhalation, P_{ALV} and flow fall exponentially and reach zero only when the respiratory system has returned to its equilibrium position. As lung volume and elastic recoil fall throughout expiration, P_{PL} also becomes less negative and gradually returns to its baseline value.

Mechanical Ventilation

Inspiration

Mechanical ventilators apply positive (supra-atmospheric) pressure to the airway. In the absence of patient effort, the pressure supplied by the ventilator (P_{AW}) during inspiration must at all times equal the sum of the pressures needed to balance elastic recoil and overcome viscous forces. During such a *passive* inflation, P_{ER} is equal to P_{ALV}, so the equation of motion becomes:

$$P_{APP} = P_{AW} = P_V + P_{ER} = P_V + P_{ALV}$$
$$P_{AW} = (R \times \dot{V}) + (\Delta V / C_{RS}) \tag{1.8}$$

Figure 1.7 shows plots of P_{AW}, P_{ALV}, P_{PL}, flow, and volume during a passive mechanical breath with constant inspiratory flow. An end-inspiratory pause is also shown, during which the delivered volume is held in the lungs for a short time before expiration begins. Since flow is constant, lung volume increases at a constant rate. If we assume that compliance doesn't change during inspiration, there must be a linear rise in P_{ALV} (which equals $\Delta V/C_{RS}$). If we also assume that resistance doesn't change, P_V(which is $R \times \dot{V}$) will also be constant. Since it is the sum of P_V and P_{ALV}, P_{AW} must also rise at a constant rate. Pleural pressure increases throughout inspiration as the lungs are inflated and the visceral and pariental pleura are forced closer together. Pleural pressure becomes positive once the chest wall exceeds its equilibrium volume. Finally, as lung volume increases, there must be a progressive rise in lung transmural pressure (i.e., the gradient between P_{ALV} and P_{PL}).

Now let's examine what happens during the end-inspiratory pause. When inspiratory flow stops and the inspired volume is held in the lungs, P_{AW} rapidly falls from its maximum or *peak pressure* (P_{PEAK}) to a so-called *plateau pressure* (P_{PLAT}). This pressure drop occurs because there are no viscous forces in the absence of gas flow, and pressure is needed only to balance the elastic recoil of the respiratory system. In other words, P_{PLAT} is simply P_{ALV} (and P_{ER}) at the end of inspiration. The difference between P_{PEAK} and P_{PLAT} must then be the pressure needed to overcome viscous forces (P_V).

In Figure 1.7, I have put pressure on the Y-axis and time on the X-axis because that's how pressure curves are shown on the ventilator interface, but it's important to recognize that the same information can be displayed using volume–pressure curves like those shown in Figure 1.3. In Figure 1.8, I have removed the curve showing lung transmural pressure (PL_{TM}) and added a curve showing the total pressure generated during a mechanical breath (P_{AW}). Since the transmural pressure of the chest wall (Pcw_{TM}) and respiratory system (PRs_{TM}) in Figure 1.3 are, in fact, P_{PL} and P_{ALV}, they have been relabeled in Figure 1.8. Later in this chapter and in several subsequent chapters, this alternative view of the pressure changes during a mechanical breath will be used

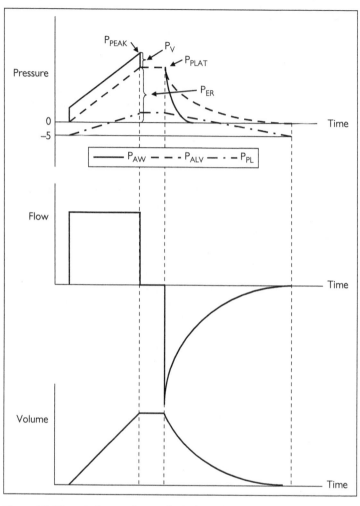

Figure 1.7 Schematic diagram of airway (P_{AW}), alveolar (P_{ALV}), and pleural (P_{PL}) pressure, flow, and volume versus time during a passive mechanical breath with constant inspiratory flow. Peak (P_{PEAK}) and plateau (P_{PLAT}) pressure and the pressure needed to balance elastic recoil (P_{ER}) and overcome viscous forces (P_V) are shown.

to examine the effect of inspiration and positive end-expiratory pressure on the change in P_{PL} and PL_{TM}.

Figure 1.9 shows how P_{AW}, P_{ALV}, P_V, and P_{ER} are affected by changes in resistance, compliance, tidal volume, and flow rate. By now, it's obvious that I like to

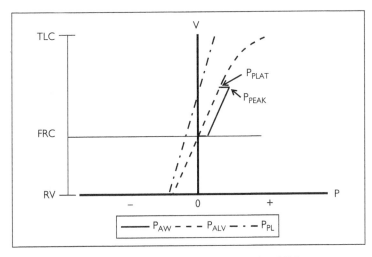

Figure 1.8 Plots of lung volume (V) versus alveolar (P_{ALV}) and pleural (P_{PL}) pressure between residual volume (RV) and total lung capacity (TLC). The total pressure supplied by the ventilator (airway pressure; P_{AW}) during passive inflation and peak (P_{PEAK}) and plateau (P_{PLAT}) pressure are also shown. Note the similarities between Figures 1.3 and 1.7.

use mechanical models, and I'm going to use another one to help you understand these pressure curves. This one consists of a balloon to represent the elastic elements of the respiratory system and a straw to simulate the airways of the lungs (Figure 1.10). Just like during mechanical ventilation, if you blow up a balloon through a straw, the pressure inside your mouth (P_M) must always equal the sum of the pressures needed to overcome the elastic recoil of the balloon (P_{ER}) and the viscous forces of the straw (P_V). In this model, P_M is analogous to P_{AW} in Equation 1.8.

Think about blowing up a balloon through a straw and look again at Equation 1.8. You would have to blow really hard (high P_M) to overcome viscous forces (P_V) if the straw were long and narrow (high R) or if you wanted to inflate the balloon very quickly (high $\dot{V}$). If you put a lot of air in the balloon (high ΔV), or if the balloon were very stiff (low C), you would need a lot of pressure to overcome elastic recoil (P_{ER}).

Now let's go back to Figure 1.9. Just like in our balloon and straw model, an increase in resistance or inspiratory flow increases P_V and P_{PEAK} without changing P_{ER} or P_{PLAT}. When compliance falls or tidal volume rises, P_{PEAK} increases with P_{ER} and P_{PLAT}, but there is no change in P_V. A decrease in resistance, flow, and volume, and an increase in compliance have just the opposite effects.

Figure 1.11 shows how a change in the *profile* of inspiratory flow affects P_{AW} and P_{ALV} when all other parameters remain constant. Since resistance doesn't change, P_V varies only with the rate of gas flow. As we saw in Figures 1.7 and 1.9,

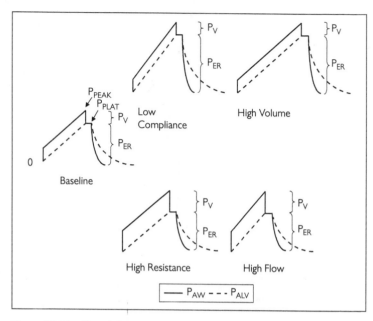

Figure 1.9 The effect of changes in compliance, resistance, volume, and flow on the pressure required to balance elastic recoil (P_{ER}) and overcome viscous forces (P_V) and on peak (P_{PEAK}) and plateau (P_{PLAT}) pressures. P_{ER} increases with a fall in compliance and an increase in tidal volume. P_V increases with resistance and flow.

if flow from the ventilator is constant (Figure 1.11A), there will be a progressive, linear rise in both P_{ALV} and P_{AW} as lung volume and elastic recoil increase, but the difference between them (P_V) won't change. If flow falls but never stops during inspiration (Figure 1.11B), P_V also falls, and P_{ALV} approaches but never equals P_{AW}. When flow is initially very rapid and falls to zero (Figure 1.11C), P_{AW} quickly reaches and then maintains its peak level. As flow decreases, P_V falls

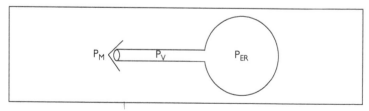

Figure 1.10 Balloon-and-straw model of the respiratory system. When inflating the balloon, the pressure in the mouth (P_M) must always equal the sum of the pressures needed to overcome viscous forces (P_V) and elastic recoil (P_{ER}).

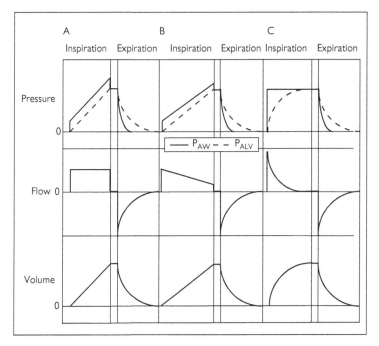

Figure 1.11 The pressure within the ventilator circuit (P_{AW}) and alveoli (P_{ALV}), flow, and volume during positive pressure mechanical breaths with three different inspiratory flow profiles.

to zero, and P_{ALV} increases in a curvilinear fashion until it equals P_{AW}. Since tidal volume and compliance don't change, P_{PLAT} is the same in Figures 1.11A, 1.11B, and 1.11C, but notice that there's a progressive fall in P_{PEAK}. That's because less and less pressure is needed as flow and P_V fall. When end-inspiratory flow is zero, P_{PEAK} equals P_{PLAT}.

Expiration

Like spontaneous breathing, expiration is normally passive during mechanical ventilation, and gas flow is driven by the stored elastic recoil of the respiratory system. As shown in Figure 1.7, flow reaches zero, and P_{ALV} and P_{PL} return to their baseline levels only when the entire tidal volume has been exhaled and the respiratory system has returned to its equilibrium position. Notice that P_{AW} reaches zero well before P_{ALV} does. The reason for this, and its importance, will be discussed in Chapters 9 and 10.

Positive End-Expiratory Pressure

Recall that the respiratory system reaches its equilibrium volume when the elastic recoil of the lungs and the chest wall are equal and opposite (Figure 1.3).

At that point, the respiratory system has no remaining elastic recoil, and P_{ALV} is zero (atmospheric pressure). Mechanical ventilators can, however, be set to increase the equilibrium volume by maintaining positive (supra-atmospheric) pressure throughout expiration. This is referred to as *positive end-expiratory pressure* (PEEP). Figure 1.12 shows that PEEP raises end-expiratory alveolar pressure, which increases P_{ALV}, P_{AW}, and P_{PL} throughout the entire mechanical breath. If we now switch to a volume–pressure curve (Figure 1.13), you can see how increasing end-expiratory alveolar pressure creates a new, higher equilibrium volume and increases end-inspiratory lung volume. PEEP is used to open or "recruit" atelectatic (collapsed) alveoli and is discussed many more times throughout this book.

Although it is usually applied intentionally, positive end-expiratory pressure can also occur as an unintended consequence of mechanical

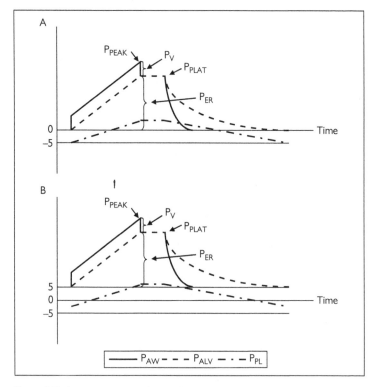

Figure 1.12 Simultaneous plots of airway (P_{AW}), alveolar (P_{ALV}), and pleural (P_{PL}) pressure versus time during a passive mechanical breath with constant inspiratory flow before (A) and after (B) the addition of 5 cmH$_2$O PEEP. Peak (P_{PEAK}) and plateau (P_{PLAT}) pressure and the pressure needed to balance elastic recoil (P_{ER}) and overcome viscous forces (P_V) are shown.

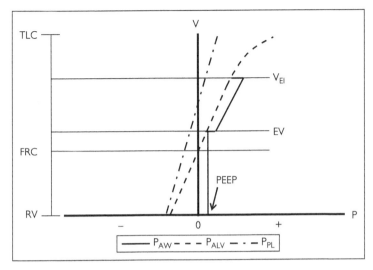

Figure 1.13 Modification of Figure 1.8 showing that PEEP (*arrow*) creates a new equilibrium volume (EV) for the respiratory system and increases end-inspiratory volume (V_{EI}).

ventilation. When the time available for expiration (expiratory time; T_E) is insufficient to allow the respiratory system to return to its equilibrium volume (with or without PEEP), flow persists at end-expiration, and elastic recoil pressure (P_{ALV}) exceeds PEEP. This additional alveolar pressure is called *intrinsic* PEEP ($PEEP_I$) to distinguish it from intentionally added *extrinsic* PEEP ($PEEP_E$). The sum of intrinsic and extrinsic PEEP is referred to as *total* PEEP ($PEEP_T$). As shown in Figure 1.14, $PEEP_I$ further increases end-inspiratory and end-expiratory lung volume, P_{AW}, P_{ALV}, and P_{PL}. Intrinsic PEEP results from a process called *dynamic hyperinflation*, which will be covered in Chapter 10.

Notice in Figures 1.12 and 1.14 that when $PEEP_E$ or $PEEP_I$ is present, P_{PLAT} is no longer equal to P_{ER}, which is the pressure needed to overcome the elastic recoil produced by the *delivered tidal volume*. Instead P_{PLAT} equals the sum of P_{ER} and $PEEP_T$, which is the *total elastic recoil pressure* of the respiratory system. This leads to an important modification of the equation of motion.

$$P_{AW} = (R_{AW} \times \dot{V}) + (\Delta V / C_{RS}) + PEEP_T \qquad (1.9)$$

Patient Effort During Mechanical Ventilation

Consider what happens when a patient makes an inspiratory effort during a mechanical breath. Now, a portion of the pressure needed for inspiration is

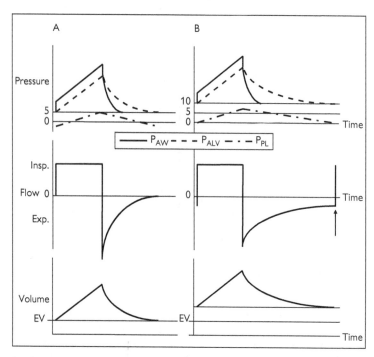

Figure 1.14 Plots of airway (P_{AW}), alveolar (P_{ALV}), and pleural (P_{PL}) pressure, flow, and volume with $PEEP_E$ of 5 cmH_2O and $PEEP_I$ of zero (A) and 5 cmH_2O (B). $PEEP_I$ occurs when there is insufficient time for complete exhalation. This is indicated by persistent flow at end-expiration (*arrow*). $PEEP_I$ further increases P_{AW}, P_{ALV}, P_{PL}, and end-inspiratory and end-expiratory lung volume. Alveolar pressure at end-expiration is the sum of $PEEP_E$ and $PEEP_I$. EV is the equilibrium volume produced by $PEEP_E$.

provided by contraction of the respiratory muscles (P_{MUS}). This means that we can rewrite the equation of motion once again:

$$P_{AW} + P_{MUS} = (R \times \dot{V}) + (\Delta V / C_{RS}) + PEEP_T \qquad (1.10)$$

$$OR \quad P_{AW} = (R \times \dot{V}) + (\Delta V / C_{RS}) + PEEP_T - P_{MUS} \qquad (1.11)$$

Equation 1.11 simply tells us that the ventilator must provide less and less positive pressure as patient effort increases. As you can probably imagine, this can have major effects on P_{AW}, P_{ALV}, P_{PL}, flow rate, and volume. The importance of patient–ventilator interactions will be discussed in several subsequent chapters.

Time Constant

Before leaving the discussion of respiratory mechanics, I want to cover one more topic, and that's the *time constant* of the respiratory system. Let's go back to the balloon and straw model of the respiratory system, but now let's imagine that the balloon is inflated and you've covered the end of the straw with your thumb. Now take your thumb away and let the air come out. It's probably easy to recognize that there are two factors that determine how fast the balloon deflates—the compliance of the balloon and the resistance of the straw.

If the elastic recoil of the balloon is high (low compliance) or the straw has a large diameter (low resistance), flow will be rapid and the balloon will empty quickly. If the balloon has little elastic recoil (high compliance) or the straw has a very small lumen (high resistance), flow will be slow, and the balloon will empty slowly.

The same is true for the respiratory system during passive expiration. In fact, it turns out that the *product* of respiratory system compliance and resistance determines how quickly expiration occurs. This is referred to as the time constant (τ) and has units of time (seconds).

$$\tau = C_{RS} \times R \tag{1.12}$$

During passive expiration, the volume of inspired gas remaining in the lungs (V) at any time (t) is determined by the inspired (tidal) volume (Vi) and the time constant.

$$V = Vi \cdot e^{-(t/\tau)} \tag{1.13}$$

In this equation, e is the base of natural logarithms (approximately 2.72) and t is the time from the start of expiration (in seconds). Fortunately, you don't have to use or even remember this equation. All you have to remember is that during a passive expiration, approximately 37%, 14%, and 5% of the tidal volume remains in the lungs after 1, 2, and 3 time constants. Because expiratory flow also decays exponentially, an identical relationship exists between the initial (maximum) flow ($\dot{V}i$) and the flow ($\dot{V}$) at any time (t) during expiration.

$$\dot{V} = \dot{V}i \cdot e^{-(t/\tau)} \tag{1.14}$$

Additional Reading

Agostoni E, Hyatt RE. Static behavior of the respiratory system. In: Macklem PT, Mead J, eds. *Handbook of Physiology: The Respiratory System*. Vol. 3, Part 1. Bethesda, MD: American Physiological Society.

Otis AB, Fenn WO, Rahn H. Mechanics of breathing in man. *J Appl Physiol*. 1950;2: 592–607.

Rodarte JR, Rehder K. Dynamics of respiration. In: Macklem PT, Mead J, eds. *Handbook of Physiology: The Respiratory System*. Vol. 3, Part 1. Bethesda, MD: American Physiological Society.

Truwitt JD, Marini JJ. Evaluation of thoracic mechanics in the ventilated patient. Part 1: primary measurements. *J Crit Care*. 1988;3:133–150.

Truwitt JD, Marini JJ. Evaluation of thoracic mechanics in the ventilated patient. Part 2: applied mechanics. *J Crit Care*. 1988;3:199–213.

Chapter 2

Gas Exchange

I use the term *gas exchange* to encompass several processes that allow the respiratory system to maintain a normal arterial partial pressure of O_2 and CO_2 (PaO_2, $PaCO_2$). Even though I separated ventilation and gas exchange in the introduction to Chapter 1, ventilation is actually an essential part of gas exchange because it delivers O_2, eliminates CO_2, and determines ventilation–perfusion ratios.

The components of normal gas exchange are:

- Delivery of oxygen
- Excretion of carbon dioxide
- Matching of ventilation and perfusion
- Gas diffusion

Before discussing each of these components, it's important to review the concept of gas partial pressure.

Partial Pressure

The *total pressure* (P_T) produced by a *gas mixture* is equal to the sum of the pressures generated by each of its components.

$$P_T = P_1 + P_2 + P_3 \ldots \tag{2.1}$$

The pressure contributed by each gas is referred to as its *partial pressure*, which is equal to total pressure multiplied by the *fractional concentration* (F) of each gas in the mixture. For example, at sea level, the total pressure of the atmosphere (barometric pressure; P_B) is 760 mmHg. Since the fractional concentration of O_2 (FO_2) in dry air is 0.21 (i.e., 21% of the gas molecules are O_2), its partial pressure (PO_2) is calculated as:

$$PO_2 = P_B \times FO_2$$
$$PO_2 = 760 \text{ mmHg} \times 0.21 = 160 \text{ mmHg} \tag{2.2}$$

Similarly, the partial pressure of nitrogen (PN_2) is 760 mmHg × 0.79, or 600 mmHg.

Partial pressure is important because O_2 and CO_2 molecules diffuse between alveolar gas and pulmonary capillary blood and between systemic capillary blood and the tissues along their partial pressure gradients, and diffusion continues until the partial pressures are equal. Gas diffusion is discussed in much more detail later in this chapter.

Delivery of Oxygen

Ventilation is responsible for delivering O_2 molecules to the alveoli, and this is the first step in transferring O_2 from outside the body to the arterial blood. As just mentioned, the PO_2 of dry air at sea level is 160 mmHg. Once gas enters the upper and lower airways, it is heated and humidified. This introduces another gas into the mixture—water. Since the partial pressure of water (P_{H2O}) at body temperature is 47 mmHg, the *inspired* partial pressure of oxygen (P_IO_2) becomes the product of FO_2 and the difference between barometric and water pressure.

$$P_IO_2 = \left(P_B - P_{H2O}\right) \times F_IO_2$$
$$P_IO_2 = \left(760 - 47\right) \times 0.21 = 150 \text{ mmHg} \tag{2.3}$$

Here, F_IO_2 is the fractional concentration of *inspired* oxygen.

When gas reaches the alveoli, the PO_2 falls even further as O_2 and CO_2 molecules are exchanged across the alveolar–capillary interface. Although there's no way to measure the mean PO_2 of the gas in all the alveoli of the lungs ($P\bar{A}O_2$), we can estimate it by using the *alveolar gas equation.*

$$P\bar{A}O_2 = [(P_B - P_{H_2O}) \times F_IO_2] - (P\bar{A}CO_2 / R) \tag{2.4}$$

This equation has two components. The first part, within the brackets, is identical to the right side of Equation 2.3 and equals the PO_2 of the gas within the conducting airways (i.e., the airways from the mouth to the terminal bronchioles). The second part equals the drop in P_IO_2 caused by the diffusion of O_2 into the capillary blood. In this portion of the equation, $P\bar{A}CO_2$ is the mean alveolar PCO_2, which is assumed to equal arterial PCO_2, and R is the ratio of CO_2 molecules entering to O_2 molecules leaving the alveolar gas. Let's assume for a moment that R is 1.0. In that case, $P\bar{A}CO_2$ would increase and $P\bar{A}O_2$ would fall by the same amount, and we could simply subtract $PaCO_2$ from P_IO_2 to get the mean alveolar PO_2. Normally, however, R is less than 1.0, and for the alveolar gas equation, it is assumed to equal 0.8. So, the decrease in PO_2 between the conducting airways and the alveoli will be $PaCO_2$ divided by 0.8 (or multiplied by 1.25). If $PaCO_2$ is 40 mmHg, we get:

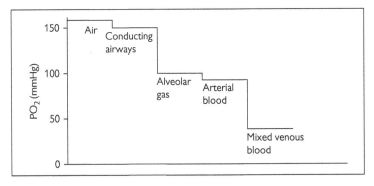

Figure 2.1 The oxygen cascade.

$$P\overline{A}O_2 = \left[(760 - 47) \times 0.21\right] - (40 / 0.8) = 150 - 50 = 100 \text{ mmHg}$$

As you can see, $P\overline{A}O_2$ varies directly with barometric pressure and F_IO_2 and inversely with $PaCO_2$. The progressive fall in PO_2 between the outside of the body and the alveoli is part of the *oxygen cascade*, which continues as O_2 enters the arterial blood and the tissues (Figure 2.1).

You can think of the calculated $P\overline{A}O_2$ as being the highest possible PaO_2 for a given P_B, F_IO_2, and $PaCO_2$. That's because the alveolar gas equation tells us what the $P\overline{A}O_2$ *and* the PaO_2 *would be* if the lungs were "perfect"—that is, if every alveolus had the same ratio of ventilation to perfusion. In fact, as you'll soon learn, there's no such thing as perfect lungs, and that's why there's always a difference between the calculated $P\overline{A}O_2$ and the measured PaO_2.

Carbon Dioxide Excretion

Carbon dioxide is a normal byproduct of cellular metabolism and continuously diffuses from the tissues into the systemic capillary blood, and from the pulmonary capillary blood into the alveolar gas. The mean alveolar and arterial PCO_2 are determined by the balance between the rates at which CO_2 is produced by the tissues ($\dot{V}_PCO_2$) and excreted by ventilation ($\dot{V}_ECO_2$).

$$PaCO_2 \propto \dot{V}_PCO_2 / \dot{V}_ECO_2 \tag{2.5}$$

If, for example, CO_2 is produced faster than it's eliminated, $PaCO_2$ will rise. If CO_2 is removed faster than it's produced, $PaCO_2$ will fall.

Although ventilation delivers O_2 and removes CO_2, not all of the gas entering and leaving the lungs takes part in this process. In fact, the *tidal volume* (V_T) can be divided into two components. The first is the *alveolar volume* (V_A), which is the portion that reaches optimally perfused alveoli and is responsible for the exchange of O_2 and CO_2. The second is referred to as the *dead space volume* (V_D) because it does not participate in gas exchange.

$$V_T = V_A + V_D \tag{2.6}$$

The total or *physiologic dead space* volume is divided into two components— airway and alveolar. The *airway dead space* is the volume of gas that remains in the conducting airways at the end of inspiration. Since this gas never reaches the alveoli, it cannot remove CO_2. *Alveolar dead space* is the volume of gas that goes to non-perfused or under-perfused alveoli, and it will be discussed later in this chapter.

If each component of Equation 2.6 is multiplied by the respiratory rate, volume is converted to volume per minute, and the relationship between the gas leaving the lungs (minute ventilation; $\dot{V}_E$), optimally perfused alveoli (alveolar ventilation; $\dot{V}_A$), and the physiologic dead space (dead space ventilation; $\dot{V}_D$) can be expressed as:

$$\dot{V}_E = \dot{V}_A + \dot{V}_D \tag{2.7}$$

Carbon dioxide excretion is directly proportional to alveolar ventilation, and this allows us to rewrite Equation 2.5 as:

$$PaCO_2 \propto \dot{V}_PCO_2 \, / \, \dot{V}_A \tag{2.8}$$

which, according to Equation 2.7, can also be written as:

$$PaCO_2 \propto \dot{V}_PCO_2 \, / \, \dot{V}_E - \dot{V}_D \tag{2.9}$$

Equation 2.9 tells us two important things. First, an increase in $PaCO_2$ (hypercapnia) can result from a drop in $\dot{V}_E$, an increase in CO_2 production, or a rise in $\dot{V}_D$. Second, any change in CO_2 production or $\dot{V}_D$ must be matched by a change in $\dot{V}_E$ if $PaCO_2$ is to remain constant.

The physiologic dead space is usually expressed as a fraction of the tidal volume (V_D/V_T). When V_D/V_T is high, V_A is low, and each breath is relatively ineffective at eliminating CO_2. When V_D/V_T is low, V_A is high, and much more

CO$_2$ is excreted. The importance of V_D/V_T can be emphasized by rewriting Equation 2.9 as:

$$PaCO_2 \propto \dot{V}_PCO_2 / \dot{V}_E \times \left(1 - V_D / V_T\right) \tag{2.10}$$

This shows that $\dot{V}_E$ must increase and decrease with V_D/V_T if PaCO$_2$ is to remain constant. Although V_D/V_T varies directly with the volume of physiologic dead space, clinically significant changes are more often due to variations in tidal volume. That is, a low V_T increases the $\dot{V}_E$ needed to maintain a given PaCO$_2$, whereas a high V_T decreases the required $\dot{V}_E$.

Matching of Ventilation and Perfusion

As shown in Figure 2.2, O$_2$ is delivered by ventilation and removed by perfusion, and CO$_2$ is delivered by perfusion and removed by ventilation. It follows that the partial pressure of oxygen and carbon dioxide in the gas of *each* alveolus (P$_A$O$_2$; P$_A$CO$_2$) must be determined by its *ratio* of ventilation to perfusion ($\dot{V}/\dot{Q}$). It's important to recognize that here P$_A$O$_2$ and P$_A$CO$_2$ refer to the partial pressure of gas in *individual alveoli*, whereas P̄AO$_2$ and P̄ACO$_2$ refer to mean values of *all* alveolar gas.

Figure 2.3 illustrates the effect of three different ventilation–perfusion ratios. An "ideal" alveolus has a $\dot{V}/\dot{Q}$ that allows the ratio of CO$_2$ to O$_2$

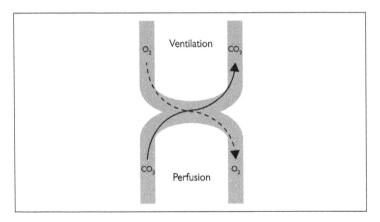

Figure 2.2 Schematic representation of gas exchange. Oxygen (O$_2$) is delivered to the gas–blood interface of the lungs by ventilation and transported to the tissues by perfusion. Carbon dioxide (CO$_2$) is transported from the tissues by perfusion and removed from the body by ventilation.

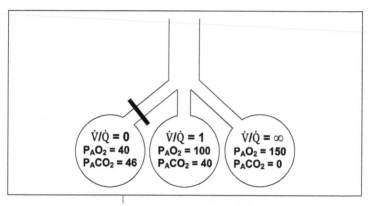

Figure 2.3 Illustration of the effect of three different ventilation–perfusion ratios ($\dot{V}/\dot{Q}$). An "ideal" alveolus has a $\dot{V}/\dot{Q}$ of about 1.0, and the alveolar gas has a partial pressure of oxygen (P_AO_2) and carbon dioxide (P_ACO_2) of approximately 100 mmHg and 40 mmHg, respectively. An alveolus with no ventilation has a $\dot{V}/\dot{Q}$ of zero, and the P_AO_2 and P_ACO_2 are the same as in the mixed venous blood. An alveolus with no perfusion has a $\dot{V}/\dot{Q}$ of infinity, and P_AO_2 and P_ACO_2 are the same as in the conducting airways.

exchange (R) to equal the ratio of total body CO_2 production to O_2 consumption (the respiratory quotient; RQ). If R and RQ are assumed to be 0.8, this ideal $\dot{V}/\dot{Q}$ is very close to 1.0, and P_AO_2 and P_ACO_2 are approximately 100 mmHg and 40 mmHg, respectively. If an alveolus receives blood flow but no ventilation, $\dot{V}/\dot{Q}$ is zero, O_2 cannot enter and CO_2 cannot leave, and the P_AO_2 and P_ACO_2 will be the same as in the mixed venous blood. If ventilation is intact but perfusion is absent, $\dot{V}/\dot{Q}$ is infinity, O_2 is not removed and CO_2 cannot enter, and the P_AO_2 and P_ACO_2 will be the same as in the conducting airways.

In fact, as shown in Figure 2.4, there is an infinite number of ventilation–perfusion ratios that may exist within individual alveoli, and every $\dot{V}/\dot{Q}$ between zero and infinity produces a unique P_AO_2 and P_ACO_2. As $\dot{V}/\dot{Q}$ increases, P_AO_2 rises and P_ACO_2 falls as ventilation delivers more O_2 and removes more CO_2. As $\dot{V}/\dot{Q}$ decreases, the opposite occurs; P_AO_2 falls and P_ACO_2 rises.

In a theoretical *perfect lung*, every alveolus has the same $\dot{V}/\dot{Q}$ and the same P_AO_2 and P_ACO_2. Normal lungs are not perfect, because they have a *distribution* of ratios representing both high and low $\dot{V}/\dot{Q}$ alveoli. This modest degree of $\dot{V}/\dot{Q}$ *mismatching* occurs because ventilation and perfusion increase at different rates from the less to the more dependent regions of the lungs. All lung diseases, regardless of whether the airways, parenchyma, or vasculature are primarily affected, generate both abnormally high and low $\dot{V}/\dot{Q}$ regions. This is because reduced ventilation or perfusion to some alveoli must be

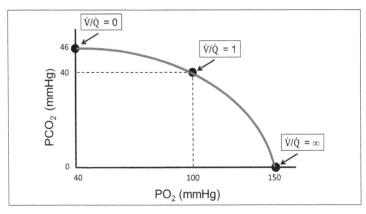

Figure 2.4 The O_2-CO_2 diagram. The line represents the PO_2 and PCO_2 of all possible ventilation–perfusion ratios ($\dot{V}/\dot{Q}$) between zero and infinity. The points representing a $\dot{V}/\dot{Q}$ of 0, 1, and infinity are shown.

accompanied by increased ventilation or perfusion to others if total ventilation and perfusion are unchanged.

Mismatching of ventilation and perfusion is important because it interferes with the ability of the respiratory system to maintain a normal PaO_2 and $PaCO_2$. You can see how and why this occurs by studying Figures 2.5 and 2.6, which show lung models that consist of two "compartments." Each compartment could represent an individual alveolus or a region of a lung that contains any number of alveoli, but for our purposes, let's assume that each is an entire lung (pretend that you're looking at a chest X-ray). The blood leaving each lung, which we'll call the pulmonary venous blood, combines to form the arterial blood.

In Figure 2.5, both lungs receive the same amount of ventilation and perfusion, so their $\dot{V}/\dot{Q}$ ratios are identical (in this case, $\dot{V}/\dot{Q}$ =1.0). Notice that under these conditions both lungs have the same P_AO_2 and pulmonary venous PO_2 (P_VO_2), and that the PO_2 and hemoglobin saturation (SO_2) of the mixed (arterial) blood are identical to those of the blood leaving each lung. Because these lungs are "perfect," the averaged alveolar and arterial PO_2 are equal, and the difference between them (the A–a gradient) is zero.

In Figure 2.6, total ventilation and perfusion are unchanged, but narrowing of the airway to the left lung has altered the $\dot{V}/\dot{Q}$ ratios. Now, the right lung receives more ventilation than perfusion ($\dot{V}/\dot{Q}$ = 1.5), and the left lung has more perfusion than ventilation ($\dot{V}/\dot{Q}$ = 0.5). As you would expect, when compared to the values in Figure 2.5, the high $\dot{V}/\dot{Q}$ of the right lung has increased P_AO_2 and P_VO_2 and lowered P_ACO_2 and pulmonary venous PCO_2 (P_VCO_2). The low $\dot{V}/\dot{Q}$ of the left lung has had the opposite effect.

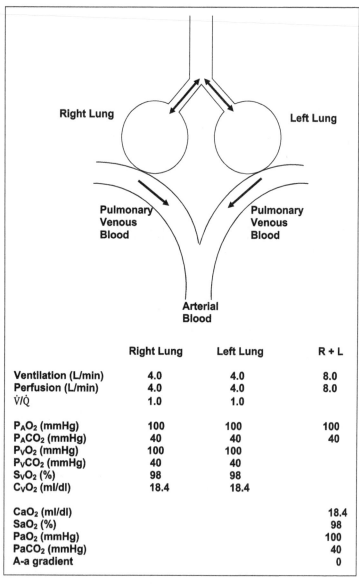

	Right Lung	Left Lung	R + L
Ventilation (L/min)	4.0	4.0	8.0
Perfusion (L/min)	4.0	4.0	8.0
$\dot{V}/\dot{Q}$	1.0	1.0	
P_AO_2 (mmHg)	100	100	100
P_ACO_2 (mmHg)	40	40	40
P_VO_2 (mmHg)	100	100	
P_VCO_2 (mmHg)	40	40	
S_VO_2 (%)	98	98	
C_VO_2 (ml/dl)	18.4	18.4	
CaO_2 (ml/dl)			18.4
SaO_2 (%)			98
PaO_2 (mmHg)			100
$PaCO_2$ (mmHg)			40
A-a gradient			0

Figure 2.5 Two-compartment model of the respiratory system. Since the lungs have identical $\dot{V}/\dot{Q}$ ratios, the arterial blood has the same PO_2 and PCO_2 as the blood leaving each lung, and the A–a gradient is zero. P_V = partial pressure of pulmonary venous blood; S_VO_2 = hemoglobin saturation of pulmonary venous blood; SaO_2 = saturation of arterial blood; C_VO_2 = O_2 content of pulmonary venous blood; CaO_2 = O_2 content of arterial blood.

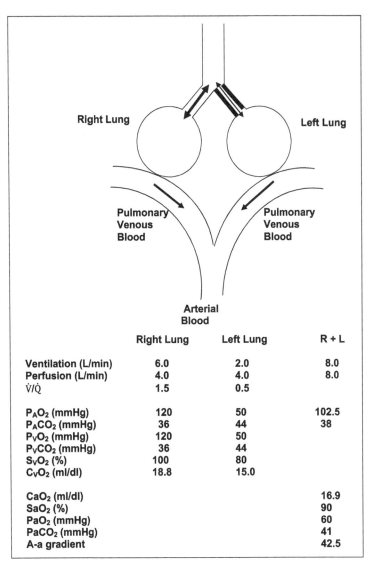

	Right Lung	Left Lung	R + L
Ventilation (L/min)	6.0	2.0	8.0
Perfusion (L/min)	4.0	4.0	8.0
$\dot{V}/\dot{Q}$	1.5	0.5	
P_AO_2 **(mmHg)**	120	50	102.5
P_ACO_2 **(mmHg)**	36	44	38
P_VO_2 **(mmHg)**	120	50	
P_VCO_2 **(mmHg)**	36	44	
S_VO_2 **(%)**	100	80	
C_VO_2 **(ml/dl)**	18.8	15.0	
CaO_2 **(ml/dl)**			16.9
SaO_2 **(%)**			90
PaO_2 **(mmHg)**			60
$PaCO_2$ **(mmHg)**			41
A-a gradient			42.5

Figure 2.6 Two-compartment model of the respiratory system. Ventilation has been diverted from the left lung to the right lung, and this has produced both low and high $\dot{V}/\dot{Q}$ ratios. Compared to Figure 2.5, the PaO_2 has fallen and the $PaCO_2$ and the A–a gradient have increased. The combined P_AO_2 and P_ACO_2 are weighted averages.

Now things really get interesting. When we combine the blood from the two lungs, we find that the PaO_2 has fallen from 100 mmHg in Figure 2.5 to 60 mmHg, and the A–a gradient has gone from 0 to 42.5. Why did this happen? To answer this question, you first need to understand that the PO_2 of a blood mixture is determined by the average *oxygen content*, not the average PO_2.

The oxygen content of blood (C_xO_2) is determined by its hemoglobin concentration (Hb) and saturation (SO_2) and is expressed as milliliters of O_2 per deciliter of blood (ml/dl).

$$C_xO_2 = 1.34 \times Hb \times SO_2 / 100 \qquad (2.11)$$

In this equation, 1.34 is the milliliters of O_2 carried by one gram of completely saturated hemoglobin (ml/g), and Hb is expressed in grams per deciliter of blood (g/dl). When we average the O_2 contents of the blood leaving the two lungs (C_VO_2) in Figure 2.6 and solve Equation 2.11 for SO_2, we find that the saturation of the arterial blood is 90%, which, based on the normal hemoglobin dissociation curve, corresponds to a PaO_2 of 60 mmHg. Since the hemoglobin concentration of the blood coming from both lungs is the same, we can actually take a shortcut and simply average the saturations rather than the O_2 contents of the pulmonary venous blood. Try it and see.

Okay, but how did $\dot{V}/\dot{Q}$ mismatching produce such a dramatic drop in the PaO_2? The explanation lies in the nonlinear shape of the hemoglobin dissociation curve. Look at Figure 2.7. If we combine two blood samples, each with a PO_2 of 80 mmHg and an SO_2 of 95%, the PO_2 and SO_2 will be unchanged in the mixture. But what if we were to decrease the PO_2 in one sample by 30 mmHg and increase it by the same amount in the other? As you can see, hemoglobin saturation (and O_2 content) is affected much more by a fall in PO_2 than by an equivalent increase. So, when we combine these blood samples, the average SO_2 is 84%, which corresponds to a PO_2 of 55 mmHg. Figure 2.7 demonstrates an essential concept: Blood from high $\dot{V}/\dot{Q}$ alveoli can never compensate for the drop in SO_2 and O_2 content caused by low $\dot{V}/\dot{Q}$ regions.

Figure 2.8 shows what happens when one lung receives no ventilation ($\dot{V}/\dot{Q} = 0$). Since no O_2 or CO_2 exchange can occur, the left lung becomes a right-to-left shunt, and mixed venous blood enters the arterial circulation. This causes an even greater fall in PaO_2 despite the higher PO_2 of the blood leaving the right lung.

What about the $PaCO_2$ in Figures 2.6 and 2.8? Just like the PaO_2, the $PaCO_2$ is determined by the average *CO2 content* of the blood coming from the two lungs. But notice that the $PaCO_2$ is actually very close to the mean PCO_2 of the pulmonary venous blood. That's because the relationship between CO_2 content and PCO_2 is nearly linear in the physiological range. This means that high $\dot{V}/\dot{Q}$ alveoli can (almost) compensate for the high CO_2 content of blood coming from low $\dot{V}/\dot{Q}$ alveoli.

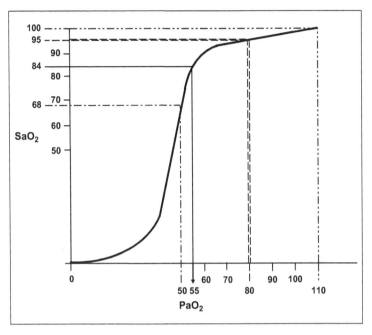

Figure 2.7 The oxygen–hemoglobin dissociation curve. When two blood samples (_ _ _ _) with a PO$_2$ of 80 mmHg and a SO$_2$ of 95% are mixed together, there is no change in the combined PO$_2$ or SO$_2$. When the PO$_2$ of one sample is reduced by 30 mmHg (_ . _ . _) and the other is increased by the same amount (_ . . _ . . _), the average SO$_2$ of the mixture (⎯⎯⎯) is only 84%, which corresponds to a PO$_2$ of 55 mmHg.

So, alveoli with low $\dot{V}/\dot{Q}$ reduce the PaO$_2$, increase the A–a gradient, and increase the PaCO$_2$. But what about high $\dot{V}/\dot{Q}$ alveoli? They, too, interfere with gas exchange because they create *alveolar dead space*. Figure 2.9 shows an extreme example in which the left lung receives ventilation but no perfusion ($\dot{V}/\dot{Q} = \infty$). Clearly, the gas entering and leaving the alveoli of this lung cannot assist with CO$_2$ excretion and is functionally no different from the gas that fills the conducting airways.

Although it may not be nearly as obvious, alveolar dead space is also produced whenever alveoli receive too little blood flow for their amount of ventilation (i.e., whenever $\dot{V}/\dot{Q} > 1$). It may help you to think of these alveoli as having *wasted ventilation* rather than dead space. For example, when an alveolus receives 10 times as much ventilation as perfusion ($\dot{V}/\dot{Q} = 10$), only 10% of the ventilation is needed to excrete CO$_2$, and the other 90% is wasted. Similarly, the right lung in Figures 2.6 and 2.8 also generates excess alveolar dead space.

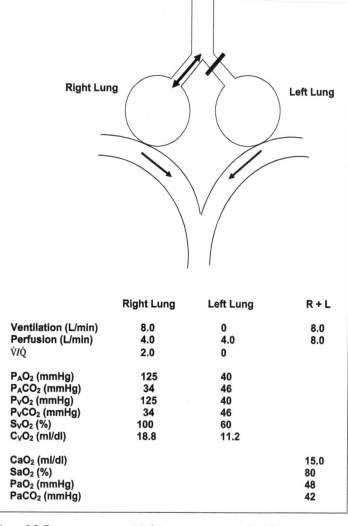

	Right Lung	Left Lung	R + L
Ventilation (L/min)	8.0	0	8.0
Perfusion (L/min)	4.0	4.0	8.0
$\dot{V}/\dot{Q}$	2.0	0	
P_AO_2 **(mmHg)**	125	40	
P_ACO_2 **(mmHg)**	34	46	
P_VO_2 **(mmHg)**	125	40	
P_VCO_2 **(mmHg)**	34	46	
S_VO_2 **(%)**	100	60	
C_VO_2 **(ml/dl)**	18.8	11.2	
CaO_2 **(ml/dl)**			15.0
SaO_2 **(%)**			80
PaO_2 **(mmHg)**			48
$PaCO_2$ **(mmHg)**			42

Figure 2.8 Two-compartment model of the respiratory system. The left lung receives no ventilation, and blood passes through it unchanged. This creates a large right-to-left intra-pulmonary shunt.

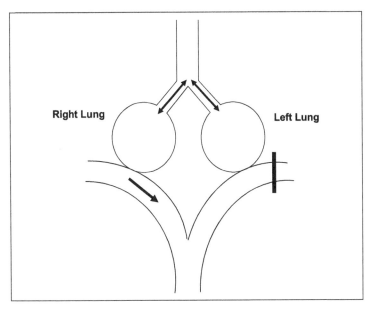

Figure 2.9 Two-compartment model of the respiratory system. The left lung receives no perfusion, so the ventilation reaching the alveoli cannot remove CO_2. This creates alveolar dead space or "wasted ventilation."

So what is the clinical effect of high $\dot{V}/\dot{Q}$ alveoli? Remember from Equations 2.8 and 2.9 that $PaCO_2$ is inversely related to alveolar ventilation, which is the difference between minute and dead space ventilation. By creating alveolar dead space, high $\dot{V}/\dot{Q}$ alveoli increase dead space ventilation and reduce alveolar ventilation, which, according to our equations, leads to an increase in $PaCO_2$.

At this point, it would seem that both high and low $\dot{V}/\dot{Q}$ alveoli can increase $PaCO_2$; but let's take a closer look. Although it may be conceptually useful to think that high $\dot{V}/\dot{Q}$ alveoli increase $PaCO_2$ through their effect on dead space ventilation, that's not really what happens. As shown in our two-compartment models, it is the alveoli with *low* $\dot{V}/\dot{Q}$ ratios that reduce CO_2 excretion and are actually responsible for any rise in the $PaCO_2$. In fact, as shown in Figures 2.6 and 2.8, blood from high $\dot{V}/\dot{Q}$ alveoli has a *low* PCO_2, and alveoli with no perfusion (Figure 2.9) contribute no blood at all to the systemic circulation.

In "real life," any rise in $PaCO_2$ resulting from $\dot{V}/\dot{Q}$ mismatching is quickly detected by central and peripheral chemoreceptors, which increase respiratory drive and minute ventilation. This is the increase in ventilation that, according to Equation 2.9, compensates for the rise in dead space ventilation and normalizes the $PaCO_2$. But, as you can see, it is triggered by the impaired CO_2 excretion of low $\dot{V}/\dot{Q}$ alveoli and actually has nothing to do with increased dead space. Furthermore, it is primarily the increase in ventilation to low $\dot{V}/\dot{Q}$ alveoli that augments CO_2 excretion (by increasing $\dot{V}/\dot{Q}$ ratios) and returns the $PaCO_2$ to normal.

Of course, our two-compartment models are a gross oversimplification. In reality, there are hundreds of millions of compartments (alveoli), each of which contributes blood with a specific content of O_2 and CO_2 that is determined by its ratio of ventilation to perfusion. The final result is the same, though. High $\dot{V}/\dot{Q}$ alveoli increase alveolar dead space and dead space ventilation, whereas low $\dot{V}/\dot{Q}$ alveoli cause a drop in the PaO_2, increase the A–a gradient, impair CO_2 excretion, and stimulate a compensatory rise in minute ventilation.

Gas Diffusion

The final component of gas exchange is the *diffusion* of O_2 and CO_2 molecules between alveolar gas and pulmonary capillary blood. During this journey, O_2 moves through the alveolar epithelium, the capillary endothelium, both basement membranes, and the plasma (where some dissolves) before entering the erythrocyte and combining with hemoglobin. Carbon dioxide molecules, of course, move in the opposite direction.

The factors that determine the rate at which gas molecules cross the alveolar–capillary interface ($\dot{V}$) are shown by this modification of Fick's law for diffusion:

$$\dot{V} \propto A \times (P_1 - P_2)/D \tag{2.12}$$

In this equation, A is the total area of contact between gas and blood in the lungs, $(P_1 - P_2)$ is the difference between the partial pressure of the gas in the alveolus and the blood, and D is the distance that the molecules must travel.

Oxygen moves from a mean P_AO_2 of around 100 mmHg to a mixed venous PO_2 of about 40 mmHg. Carbon dioxide diffuses from a mixed venous PCO_2 of about 46 mmHg to a P_ACO_2 of approximately 40 mmHg. Remember, though, that the actual PO_2 and PCO_2 of the gas in each alveolus are determined by its $\dot{V}/\dot{Q}$ ratio.

The lungs have an enormous gas–blood interface of approximately 100 square meters, and the alveolar-capillary membrane is incredibly thin at 0.2–0.5 μm. So it's not surprising that O_2 and CO_2 normally equilibrate very rapidly between alveolar gas and capillary blood. It's estimated that blood normally spends about 0.75 second in each alveolar capillary. But, as shown in Figure 2.10A, it normally takes only about one-third of this time for the alveolar and capillary PO_2 and PCO_2 to equilibrate. Even during exercise, when transit time is reduced by the increase in cardiac output, equilibration occurs before blood leaves the alveoli.

Diseases that decrease the area of the gas–blood interface or increase diffusion distance, however, slow the rate of diffusion. If diffusion impairment is severe (Figure 2.10B), there may be insufficient time for equilibration to occur, and this will produce a gradient between alveolar and end-capillary PO_2 and PCO_2. As you can see from Figure 2.10, because of the larger partial pressure gradient, the PaO_2 will be affected much more than the $PaCO_2$. If diffusion impairment does cause the $PaCO_2$ to rise, a compensatory increase in minute ventilation will be needed to return it to normal.

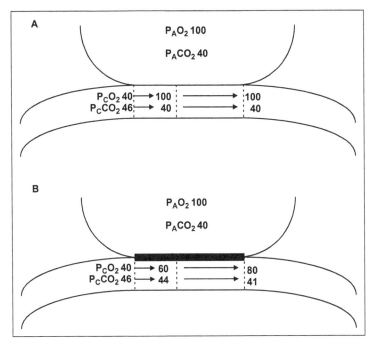

Figure 2.10 (A) The partial pressure of O_2 and CO_2 in the capillary blood entering an alveolus (PcO_2, $PcCO_2$) normally equilibrates with alveolar gas (P_AO_2, P_ACO_2) within the first third of its transit time. (B) When there is a loss of blood–gas interface or an increase in the diffusion distance (represented by the thick line), there may be insufficient time for equilibration to occur.

Additional Reading

Petersson J, Glenny RW. Gas exchange and ventilation–perfusion relationships in the lung. *Eur Respir J.* 2014;44:1023–1041.

Wagner PD. The physiological basis of pulmonary gas exchange: Implications for clinical interpretation of arterial blood gases. *Eur Respir J.* 2015;45:227–243.

Chapter 3

Cardiovascular–Pulmonary Interactions

The heart, great vessels, pulmonary circulation, and a portion of the systemic circulation are constantly exposed to non-atmospheric pressures. Figure 3.1 shows that the cardiovascular system can be divided into several "compartments" based on the prevailing external (extramural) pressure. Within the thorax, the visceral pleura completely surrounds both lungs, and the parietal pleura lines the chest wall, the diaphragm, and the mediastinum. It follows that the heart, aorta, superior vena cava, and pulmonary arteries and veins are constantly exposed to pleural pressure (P_{PL}). On the other hand, alveolar pressure (P_{ALV}) is the external pressure on the pulmonary capillaries, which run through the walls of the alveoli. The blood vessels within the abdominal compartment are exposed to intra-abdominal pressure (P_{AB}), while the extramural pressure on all other systemic vessels is atmospheric pressure (P_{ATM}).

   These external pressures are generated solely or in part by the respiratory system and continuously change during spontaneous and mechanical ventilation. Since these pressures directly alter the internal (intramural) and transmural pressures of the heart chambers and systemic and pulmonary blood vessels, ventilation can have an enormous impact on cardiac and circulatory function. That's why it's so important for physicians who care for critically ill, mechanically ventilated patients to understand the interactions that occur between the pulmonary and cardiovascular systems. I will begin by reviewing certain aspects of normal cardiovascular physiology.

Essential Cardiovascular Physiology

Intramural, Extramural, and Transmural Pressure

As discussed in Chapter 1, the pressure inside a gas-filled (or liquid-filled) elastic structure is called the *intramural pressure* (P_{IM}), and the external pressure is referred to as the *extramural pressure* (P_{EM}). The pressure gradient across the wall of the structure is called the *transmural pressure* (P_{TM}), which is calculated by subtracting the extramural from the intramural pressure.

$$P_{TM} = P_{IM} - P_{EM} \tag{3.1}$$

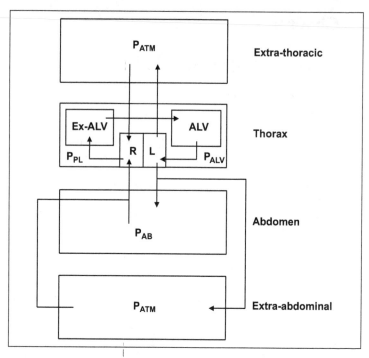

Figure 3.1 The model divides the circulatory system into four "compartments" based on location and extramural pressure. Within the thorax, the right (R) and left (L) atria and ventricles, superior vena cava, aorta, and extra-alveolar (Ex-ALV) pulmonary vessels (arteries and veins) are exposed to pleural pressure (P_{PL}), while the alveolar (ALV) vessels (pulmonary capillaries) are exposed to alveolar pressure (P_{ALV}). Systemic vessels within the abdominal compartment are exposed to intra-abdominal pressure (P_{AB}). Upper body non-thoracic and lower body non-abdominal vessels are exposed to atmospheric pressure (P_{ATM}).

The main thing I want you to remember is that intramural pressures within a tube or circuit determine the rate and direction of flow, whereas the transmural pressure of an elastic structure determines its volume. In Chapter 1, we applied these principles when talking about the pressure needed to overcome viscous forces and elastic recoil during ventilation. In this chapter, we will use them to explain changes in blood flow between two portions of the circulatory system and changes in the volume and size of the heart chambers.

Before we move on, I want to remind you that any change in the extramural pressure of an elastic structure has a direct effect on its intramural pressure. For example, if you squeeze an inflated balloon, intramural and extramural pressure increase by the same amount. Similarly, changes in pleural, alveolar, and intra-abdominal pressure alter the pressure within the heart and the intra-thoracic and intra-abdominal blood vessels.

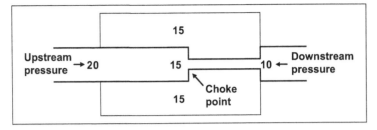

Figure 3.2 The "waterfall effect" occurs when upstream intravascular pressure exceeds, and downstream pressure is less than, extramural pressure. As intravascular pressure falls during blood flow, the vessel will narrow once transmural pressure becomes negative. This produces a choke point, and flow is then determined by the gradient between upstream pressure and the pressure at the choke point.

Blood Flow and Waterfalls

Like gas flow, blood flow can occur only by overcoming viscous forces, and this causes a progressive fall in intramural (intravascular) pressure. Consider what happens when intravascular pressure initially exceeds but then falls below extramural pressure (Figure 3.2). Once this occurs, the vessel will collapse when a critical negative transmural (closing) pressure has been reached. Since veins and capillaries have little structural rigidity, they collapse shortly after transmural pressure becomes negative, and flow then stops. When this happens, though, the intramural pressure gradient disappears, the pressure within the collapsed segment equals the upstream driving pressure, the vessel opens, and flow resumes. But as soon as flow starts, intramural pressure falls and the vessel collapses. Of course, this vicious cycle doesn't really happen. Instead, an equilibrium is reached in which the capillary or vein narrows but flow persists. Under these conditions, the pressure gradient driving flow is no longer the difference between the upstream and downstream ends of the vessel, but rather the difference between the upstream pressure and the pressure at the so-called choke point (which is just slightly less than extramural pressure).

It's especially fitting to use the terms "upstream" and "downstream" because this situation is often compared to a waterfall. In Figure 3.3, the vertical distance between the upstream part of the river and the river below the waterfall represents the pressure gradient between the two ends of the blood vessel, while the top of the waterfall is analogous to the pressure at the choke point. If you think about it, you'll see that the rate at which water rushes over the falls depends only on the vertical distance between the upstream portion of the river and the top of the waterfall (i.e., the slope of the riverbed). Just like the difference between the pressure at the choke point and downstream pressure in Figure 3.2 does not influence flow through the vessel, the height of the waterfall has no effect on how fast water flows over it. We will be talking a lot more about this *waterfall effect* throughout the rest of this chapter.

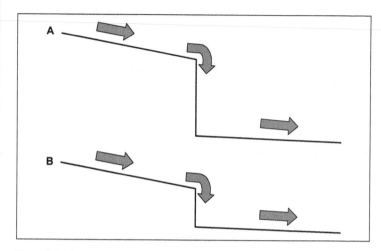

Figure 3.3 The rate at which water flows over a waterfall depends only on the slope of the river bed and is not affected by the height of the waterfall.

Cardiac Output and Stroke Volume

Cardiac output (CO) is equal to the product of heart rate (HR) and stroke volume (SV).

$$CO = HR \times SV \qquad (3.2)$$

Stroke volume is determined by the interaction of three factors:

- Ventricular preload
- Ventricular afterload
- Ventricular contractility

Preload

Technically, *preload* is the length of the cardiac myocytes just before the ventricle contracts. Starling's law tells us that, up to a point, the force of contraction increases with muscle cell length. Since we can't measure the actual preload, ventricular volume at end-diastole is the most appropriate substitute. In clinical practice, however, we typically use end-diastolic pressure (EDP), which is related to end-diastolic volume (EDV) by ventricular compliance. Figure 3.4 is a *ventricular function curve* that shows the relationship between EDV and SV. Note that this curve has two parts—an *ascending portion* where SV varies significantly with preload, and a *plateau* where changes in preload have little effect on SV.

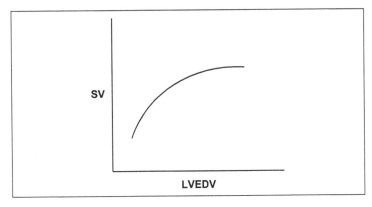

Figure 3.4 The relationship between left ventricular end-diastolic volume (LVEDV) and the stroke volume (SV) generated during ventricular contraction. As muscle length and ventricular volume increase, contractile force and SV rapidly increase, then plateau.

There are three determinants of ventricular preload:

- The rate at which blood enters the right atrium from the systemic veins (venous return)
- Ventricular compliance
- The duration of diastole, which is the time available for ventricular filling

Let's take a closer look at the first two.

Venous Return

If we rearrange the equation used to calculate resistance in Chapter 1 (Equation 1.3), you can see that flow equals the intramural pressure gradient divided by resistance.

$$\dot{V} = \Delta P_{IM}/R \tag{3.3}$$

We can use this equation to examine the factors that determine the rate at which blood returns to the right atrium (RA). Here, $\dot{V}$ is the venous return, ΔP_{IM} is the difference between *mean systemic pressure* (MSP) and right atrial intramural pressure ($P_{RA_{IM}}$), and R is the resistance of the veins returning blood to the heart. The mean systemic pressure is determined only by the compliance of the systemic arteries and veins and the volume of blood they contain. In research studies, it is assumed to be the intravascular pressure during cardiac arrest.

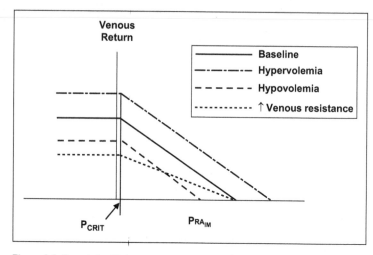

Figure 3.5 The relationship between venous return and intramural right atrial pressure (PRA_{IM}). As PRA_{IM} falls, venous return steadily increases, then plateaus once the critical pressure (P_{CRIT}) has been reached. P_{CRIT} is normally very close to atmospheric pressure. Mean systemic pressure and venous return at a given PRA_{IM} vary directly with intravascular volume. Increased venous resistance reduces the slope of the curve and decreases maximum venous return.

Guyton and colleagues were the first to construct *venous return curves* (Figure 3.5). As expected, venous return increases as PRA_{IM} falls and the pressure gradient driving flow increases. Note that venous return stops when the curve intersects the *x*-axis; this is when PRA_{IM} equals MSP. Also notice that venous return does not increase indefinitely as PRA_{IM} falls; instead, it plateaus at a so-called *critical pressure*. As you may have guessed, this plateau, in spite of further decreases in downstream pressure, is due to a waterfall effect.

The extramural pressure of the jugular and axillary veins, which drain the head, neck, and arms, is P_{ATM}, whereas the inferior vena cava (IVC) is exposed to P_{AB}. Since PRA_{IM} is the downstream pressure for both, a waterfall effect is created as soon as PRA_{IM} (and intramural venous pressure) falls below P_{ATM} or P_{AB}. The back pressure for blood flow from the upper and lower body then becomes P_{ATM} and P_{AB}, respectively, and further decreases in PRA_{IM} cannot increase venous return.

Figure 3.5 also illustrates that venous return depends on intravascular volume through its effect on MSP. Hypovolemia reduces MSP and the pressure gradient driving venous return. Volume loading increases MSP and venous return. Also note that increasing venous resistance reduces maximum venous return and decreases the slope of the venous return curve.

Ventricular Compliance

During diastole, blood flow from the atria to the ventricles is directly related to the pressure gradient between them (Equation 3.3). Also, if we rearrange the compliance equation from Chapter 1 (Equation 1.2), you can see that the volume of blood entering the ventricles is proportional to ventricular compliance and the change in ventricular transmural pressure:

$$\Delta V = \Delta P_{TM} \times C \qquad (3.4)$$

If ventricular compliance is low (i.e., the ventricle is stiff), intramural and transmural pressure rise rapidly during diastole, the pressure gradient quickly disappears, flow stops, and there is relatively little ventricular filling (Figure 3.6). This means that a ventricle with low compliance will have relatively little end-diastolic volume (preload) for a given end-diastolic pressure. If ventricular compliance is high, much more blood can enter before pressure equalizes, and preload will be relatively high at the same end-diastolic pressure.

Ventricular compliance can be altered by a number of factors, including hypertrophy, ischemia, and infiltrative diseases, but for this discussion, I want to focus on the effect of the normal pericardium. Because it is relatively non-compliant, the pericardium limits the total volume of blood that the ventricles can hold. So, if the end-diastolic volume of one ventricle increases, the interventricular septum shifts toward the other ventricle, thereby reducing its compliance, diastolic filling, and preload. This is referred to as *ventricular interdependence*. As you'll see later in this chapter, reciprocal changes in the volume within the right (RV) and left (LV) ventricles normally occur during the

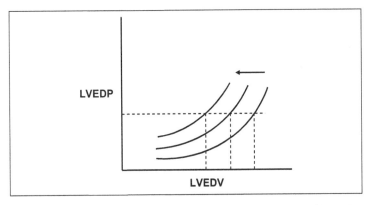

Figure 3.6 The relationship between left ventricular end-diastolic pressure (LVEDP) and volume (LVEDV). As ventricular compliance falls (*arrow*), progressively less blood enters the ventricle at the same intraventricular pressure (*dashed lines*).

respiratory cycle. *Abnormal ventricular interdependence* occurs when this effect is exaggerated by pericardial or myocardial disease.

Afterload

Ventricular afterload is defined as the wall stress generated during systole. Wall stress (σ) is proportional to the intramural pressure needed to eject blood (P_{IM}) and the internal ventricular radius (r), and inversely related to the thickness of the ventricle (T).

$$\sigma \propto (P_{IM} \times r) / T \tag{3.5}$$

From a practical standpoint, it's much easier to forget about ventricular radius and thickness (which you won't know anyway) and simply remember that LV and RV afterload are directly proportional to mean systemic arterial ($P\overline{SA}_{IM}$) and mean pulmonary arterial ($P\overline{PA}_{IM}$) pressure, respectively. But, what determines these pressures? Well, if we rearrange Equation 3.3 and make a few substitutions, you can see that LV and RV afterload are also directly related to cardiac output and systemic (SVR) and pulmonary (PVR) vascular resistance, respectively.

$$\text{LV afterload} \propto P\overline{SA}_{IM} \propto (CO \times SVR) \tag{3.6}$$

$$\text{RV afterload} \propto P\overline{PA}_{IM} \propto (CO \times PVR) \tag{3.7}$$

Since the pulmonary circulation is a low-pressure, low-resistance circuit, RV afterload is normally low, and ventricular contraction must produce only a

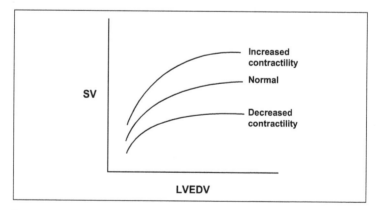

Figure 3.7 A series of ventricular function curves showing the effect of changes in contractility on the relationship between stroke volume (SV) and left ventricular end-diastolic volume (LVEDV).

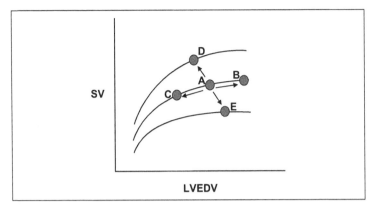

Figure 3.8 A change in preload increases (A → B) or decreases (A → C) stroke volume (SV) along one ventricular function curve. A reduction in afterload or an increase in contractility (A → D) increases SV while reducing left ventricular end-diastolic volume (LVEDV). Decreased contractility or an increase in afterload (A → E) reduces SV and increases LVEDV.

small amount of intramural pressure. The LV must generate much more pressure during systole because systemic blood pressure and vascular resistance are much higher, and afterload is proportionally increased.

Contractility

Ventricular contractility is the inherent ability of the ventricle to generate pressure during systole, and it's reduced by any disease that damages the myocardium. As shown in Figure 3.7, differences in contractility are commonly represented by a series of ventricular function curves.

The Interaction of Preload, Afterload, and Contractility

Figure 3.8 shows how SV and LV end-diastolic volume are affected by changes in preload, afterload, and contractility. As you've already seen (Figure 3.4), changes in preload move stroke volume along a single curve. Increasing contractility or decreasing afterload shifts the curve upward and to the left, meaning that SV rises and end-diastolic volume falls. A decrease in contractility or an increase in afterload shifts the curve downward and to the right, thereby reducing SV and increasing end-diastolic volume.

Spontaneous Ventilation and Cardiovascular Function

The changes in P_{PL}, P_{ALV}, P_{AB}, and lung transmural pressure (PL_{TM}) during a spontaneous breath are shown in Figure 3.9. As discussed in Chapter 1, P_{PL} is normally negative (sub-atmospheric) at end-expiration. As the inspiratory

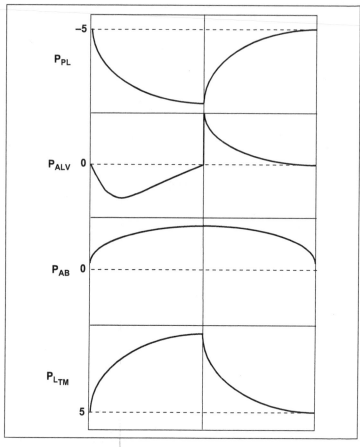

Figure 3.9 Schematic representation of the changes in pleural pressure (P_{PL}), alveolar pressure (P_{ALV}), intra-abdominal pressure (P_{AB}), and lung transmural pressure (PL_{TM}) during spontaneous breathing. Insp = inspiration; Exp = expiration

muscles expand the chest wall, lung volume and elastic recoil increase. This causes a progressive drop in P_{PL}, which reaches its lowest (most negative) value at the end of inspiration. Alveolar pressure is zero (atmospheric pressure) at end-expiration. During inspiration, P_{ALV} becomes negative as the lungs expand. This generates the pressure gradient between P_{ALV} and pressure at the mouth (P_{ATM}) that drives air into the lungs. As the lungs fill, P_{ALV} rises and returns to zero at end-inspiration. Lung transmural pressure is the pressure acting on the lungs. It equals P_{ALV} minus P_{PL}, and the rise in PL_{TM} during inspiration is what drives the increase in lung volume. Since P_{ALV} is zero (atmospheric pressure) at both the beginning and the end of inspiration (Figure 3.9), the rise in $P_{L_{TM}}$ is due to the fall in P_{PL}. As the lungs expand and the diaphragm descends, intra-abdominal volume decreases, which raises P_{AB}.

During relaxed (passive) expiration, $P_{L_{TM}}$ falls with lung volume, and P_{PL} and P_{AB} return to baseline levels. The elastic recoil generated during inspiration increases P_{ALV}, which drives gas from the lungs. Alveolar pressure and expiratory flow reach zero once the respiratory system has returned to its equilibrium volume. Based on our previous discussion, these pressure changes have predictable effects on RV and LV preload, afterload, and stroke volume (Figure 3.10).

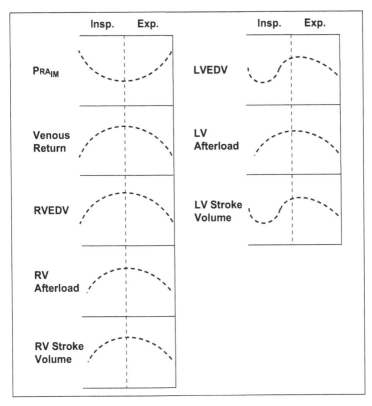

Figure 3.10 Schematic representation of the hemodynamic changes that occur during spontaneous ventilation. Insp = inspiration; Exp = expiration; $P_{RA_{IM}}$ = intramural right atrial pressure; RVEDV = right ventricular end-diastolic volume; LVEDV = left ventricular end-diastolic volume

The Effect on RV Preload

Since changes in pleural pressure cause a similar change in the pressures within the heart chambers, the drop in P_{PL} reduces $P_{RA_{IM}}$, which increases the pressure gradient driving venous return. Increased venous return augments RV filling and preload. Usually, this outweighs the increase in RV afterload (see The Effect on Pulmonary Vascular Resistance and RV Afterload), and RV stroke volume rises. Passive expiration reverses these hemodynamic changes, and venous return, RV end-diastolic volume, and RV stroke volume fall as P_{PL} returns to its baseline level.

The Effect on LV Preload

Due to ventricular interdependence, the increase in RV volume reduces LV compliance and decreases diastolic filling. This reduces LV preload and stroke volume at the beginning of inspiration. Subsequently, increased RV stroke volume augments LV preload sufficiently to overcome the rise in LV afterload (see The Effect on LV Afterload), and LV stroke volume increases.

During expiration, LV preload and stroke volume transiently rise with the decrease in RV volume and improved LV diastolic filling but then fall due to the reduction in RV stroke volume.

The Effect on Pulmonary Vascular Resistance and RV Afterload

Recall that the pulmonary vasculature can be divided into two "compartments" based on the prevailing extramural pressure (Figure 3.1). The pulmonary capillaries are often referred to as *alveolar vessels* because they are exposed to alveolar pressure. The pulmonary arteries and veins are *extra-alveolar* and are exposed to pleural pressure.

Alveolar Vessels

The transmural pressure of the pulmonary capillaries (Pc_{TM}) is the difference between capillary intramural pressure (Pc_{IM}) and alveolar pressure (P_{ALV}).

$$Pc_{TM} = Pc_{IM} - P_{ALV} \tag{3.8}$$

In turn, capillary intramural pressure depends on the location of each vessel relative to the left atrium.

At this point, it's important to recall that a column of water (or blood) generates *hydrostatic pressure*. If you fill a 30-centimeter-long tube with water and hold it vertically, the pressure at the bottom will exceed the pressure at the top by 30 cmH_2O. Similarly, when standing, the pressure inside the veins of the feet exceeds the pressure in the femoral veins by 1 cmH_2O for every centimeter of vertical distance between them.

There is normally a continuous column of blood between the pulmonary capillaries and the left atrium. Since pulmonary venous resistance is very low, Pc_{IM} will be almost identical to intramural left atrial pressure ($P_{LA_{IM}}$) *when they are at the same vertical height in the thorax.* Hydrostatic pressure progressively increases and decreases Pc_{IM} by 1.0 cmH$_2$O (0.74 mmHg) respectively, for every centimeter that the vessel is below or above the left atrial level.

We can consider P_{ALV} to be uniform throughout the lungs. Since Pc_{IM} varies with hydrostatic pressure, capillary transmural pressure and volume must decrease from the dependent to the non-dependent portions of the lungs. In 1964, West and colleagues famously divided the lungs into three "zones" based on the relationship between mean pulmonary artery pressure ($P\overline{PA}_{IM}$), Pc_{IM}, and P_{ALV} (Figure 3.11).

In the most dependent region (Zone 3), $P\overline{PA}_{IM}$ is greater than Pc_{IM}, which exceeds P_{ALV}. Since capillary transmural pressure is positive throughout, the capillaries are filled with blood, their resistance is low, and flow is driven by the difference between $P\overline{PA}_{IM}$ and $P_{LA_{IM}}$. As hydrostatic pressure increases from the top to the bottom of Zone 3, $P\overline{PA}_{IM}$ (which is also affected by hydrostatic pressure) and Pc_{IM} increase, transmural capillary pressure rises, the capillaries dilate, resistance falls, and blood flow increases.

In Zone 1, the capillaries are far above the left atrial level, and both $P\overline{PA}_{IM}$ and Pc_{IM} are less than P_{ALV}. This means that transmural pressure is negative along the entire length of the capillaries, which are collapsed and empty, and no flow occurs.

In Zone 2, P_{ALV} is greater than Pc_{IM} but less than $P\overline{PA}_{IM}$. This produces a waterfall effect, in which capillary flow is determined by the gradient between $P\overline{PA}_{IM}$ and P_{ALV} and is independent of Pc_{IM} and $P_{LA_{IM}}$. Like in Zone 3, capillary resistance

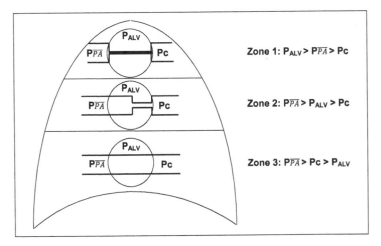

Figure 3.11 West's zones of the lung are based on the relationship between mean pulmonary artery pressure P$\overline{PA}$, intramural capillary pressure (Pc), and alveolar pressure (P$_{ALV}$). In Zone 1, the capillaries are collapsed, and no flow occurs. Vessel resistance decreases and blood flow increases from the top of Zone 2 to the bottom of Zone 3.

falls and flow increases from the top to the bottom of Zone 2 as both $P\overline{PA}_{IM}$ and Pc_{IM} increase.

Based on this discussion, you can see that the overall resistance of the alveolar vessels increases with the number of capillaries in Zones 1 and 2.

Extra-alveolar Vessels

The transmural pressure of the pulmonary arteries and veins is the difference between intramural pressure and P_{PL}. Unlike in other blood vessels, though, transmural pressure does not determine the radius and volume of the extra-alveolar vessels. That's because the pulmonary arteries and veins are attached to the lung parenchyma, which provides outward *radial traction*. In this way, the extra-alveolar vessels are just like the bronchioles, which are pulled open by the "tethering effect" of the lung parenchyma.

Lung Volume and Pulmonary Vascular Resistance

Recall from our previous discussion that, during a spontaneous breath, the rise in $P_{L_{TM}}$ is due solely to the drop in P_{PL}. Since the left atrium is exposed to P_{PL}, $P_{LA_{IM}}$ also falls, which reduces both intramural and transmural capillary pressure. This narrows the alveolar vessels, increases their resistance, and increases the number of capillaries in Zones 1 and 2. At the same time, the increase in elastic recoil that accompanies lung inflation augments the outward traction on the extra-alveolar vessels, which increases their diameter and reduces their resistance. As shown in Figure 3.12, total pulmonary vascular resistance (the sum of alveolar and extra-alveolar resistance) and RV afterload are normally

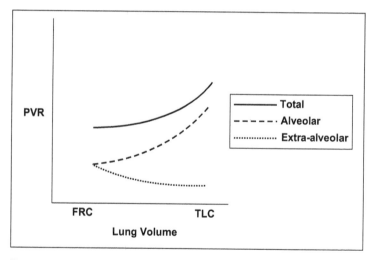

Figure 3.12 The change in pulmonary vascular resistance (PVR) between functional residual capacity (FRC) and total lung capacity (TLC). Total PVR is the sum of the resistance of the alveolar and extra-alveolar vessels.

lowest in the tidal volume range and progressively increase between functional residual capacity and total lung capacity.

The Effect on LV Afterload

The fall in P_{PL} during inspiration reduces LV end-diastolic pressure, but since most of the arterial circulation is outside the thorax, there's no change in mean arterial pressure. It follows that the LV must generate more pressure to eject blood during systole, and its afterload increases. Left ventricular afterload falls during expiration as P_{PL} returns to baseline.

Factors Affecting the Magnitude of Hemodynamic Changes

The hemodynamic effects produced by a spontaneous breath depend on three factors:

- The magnitude of the fall in P_{PL}
- The magnitude of the rise in $P_{L_{TM}}$
- Baseline ventricular function

Pleural Pressure

The magnitude of the fall in P_{PL} during inspiration varies directly with lung volume, airway resistance, and inspiratory flow, and inversely with lung compliance. In other words, P_{PL} becomes more negative with large, rapid breaths, when airway resistance is high, and when the lungs are stiff. Within the limits imposed by the critical pressure (Figure 3.5), the greater the fall in P_{PL}, the greater the increase in venous return, RV and LV preload, and LV afterload.

Lung Transmural Pressure

Because it is due to the fall in P_{PL}, the magnitude of the increase in $P_{L_{TM}}$ during a spontaneous breath also varies directly with tidal volume, airway resistance, and inspiratory flow, and inversely with lung compliance. The greater the rise in $P_{L_{TM}}$, the greater the increase in capillary and total pulmonary vascular resistance and RV afterload.

Ventricular Function

The extent to which changes in ventricular preload alter LV stroke volume and blood pressure depends primarily on baseline LV preload (Figure 3.13). If preload is already high, an increase in LV end-diastolic volume will have little effect on stroke volume and blood pressure. If however, LV preload is low, the shape of the curve dictates that even a small increase in end-diastolic volume will significantly augment stroke volume. This leads to a characteristic, cyclical change in blood pressure in hypovolemic, "volume-responsive" patients.

As shown in Figure 3.14, the transient drop in LV preload and stroke volume early in inspiration causes blood pressure to fall. From mid-inspiration to early expiration, blood pressure rises with the increase in LV preload and stroke volume. Between mid-expiration and early inspiration, blood pressure decreases with the drop in LV stroke volume.

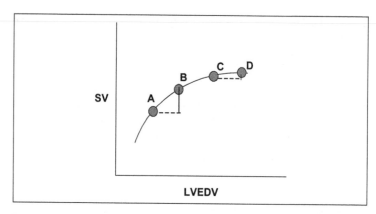

Figure 3.13 When left ventricular end-diastolic volume (LVEDV) and stroke volume (SV) occupy a point on the ascending portion of the ventricular function curve, the increase in LV preload produced by a spontaneous breath (*dashed line*) will cause a relatively large rise in SV (A → B). When ventricular preload is high, the increase in LVEDV has little effect on SV (C → D).

Spontaneous Ventilation and the Cardiovascular System: Take-Home Points

- Spontaneous ventilation causes a cyclical decrease in P_{PL}, which increases venous return, RV and LV preload, and LV afterload, and a cyclical rise in PL_{TM}, which increases PVR and RV afterload.
- The hemodynamic significance of these changes depends on the magnitude of the change in P_{PL} and PL_{TM} and on baseline ventricular function:
  - The change in P_{PL} and PL_{TM} varies directly with tidal volume, airway resistance, and inspiratory flow, and inversely with lung compliance.
  - The hemodynamic effect of a fall in P_{PL} is greater in patients with low baseline LV preload.

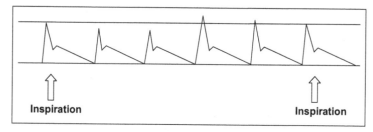

Figure 3.14 The variation in arterial blood pressure during spontaneous ventilation when LV preload is low.

Mechanical Ventilation and Cardiovascular Function

The pressure changes occurring during a *passive* (no patient effort) mechanical breath with constant inspiratory flow are shown in Figure 3.15A. Since atmospheric pressure is considered to be zero, the transmural pressure of the respiratory system ($P_{ALV} - P_{ATM}$) is simply P_{ALV}, which increases linearly with lung volume. The gradient between the pressure in the ventilator circuit (airway pressure; P_{AW}) and P_{ALV} overcomes viscous forces and drives gas through the airways. Pleural pressure rises (becomes less negative) as the visceral pleura is forced outward against the parietal pleura, and reaches zero when the respiratory system expands to the equilibrium volume of the chest wall. Above this volume, the elastic recoil of the chest wall is directed inward, the parietal pleura is pushed against the visceral pleura of the expanding lungs, and P_{PL} becomes positive (supra-atmospheric). The volume increase during inspiration is driven by the rise in PL_{TM}. We saw that during a spontaneous breath, this is due solely to the fall in P_{PL}. During mechanical inflation, PL_{TM} increases because P_{ALV} rises out of proportion to P_{PL}. As the thorax expands and the diaphragm is pushed into the abdominal compartment, P_{AB} increases by about the same amount as P_{PL}.

During passive expiration, P_{AW} immediately returns to the level of extrinsic PEEP ($PEEP_E$), and the gradient between P_{ALV} and $PEEP_E$ drives gas from the lungs. Alveolar pressure and PL_{TM} fall with elastic recoil and lung volume, and expiratory flow stops when P_{ALV} equals $PEEP_E$. Pleural pressure and P_{AB} decrease with lung volume and return to their baseline levels at end-expiration.

Now look at Figure 3.15B. You were introduced to this alternative way of representing pressure changes in Chapter 1. It has the same information as Figure 3.15A, but I'm reintroducing the concept of volume–pressure curves because it will be easier to see how changes in tidal volume and compliance affect P_{PL} and PL_{TM}.

The hemodynamic effects of a mechanical breath are shown in Figure 3.16. Note that, for the most part, they are the opposite of those occurring during spontaneous breathing.

The Effect on RV and LV Preload

During mechanical inflation, the rise in P_{PL} causes $P_{RA_{IM}}$ to increase, which reduces venous return and RV filling. The drop in RV preload and increase in RV afterload (see The Effect on RV Afterload) reduces RV stroke volume.

The decrease in RV end-diastolic volume transiently increases LV compliance, preload, and stroke volume, but, despite the drop in afterload (see The Effect on LV Afterload), LV stroke volume then falls with RV stroke volume.

Passive expiration reverses these hemodynamic changes. Venous return increases, which augments RV preload and stroke volume. LV preload and

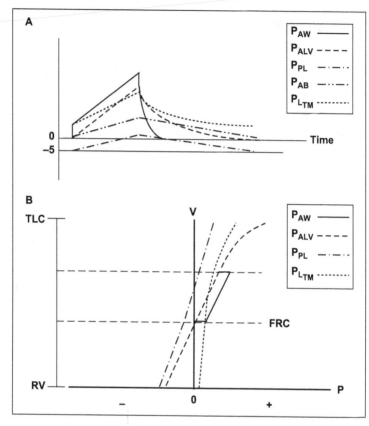

Figure 3.15 The change in airway (P_{AW}), alveolar (P_{ALV}), pleural (P_{PL}), lung transmural ($P_{L_{TM}}$), and abdominal (P_{AB}) pressure during a mechanical breath shown as (A) pressure–time curves and (B) volume–pressure curves.

stroke volume initially fall with the increase in RV filling but then increase due to the rise in venous return and RV stroke volume.

The Effect on RV Afterload

Alveolar pressure normally increases more than P_{PL} during mechanical inflation (Figure 3.15). Since $P_{LA_{IM}}$ and P_{PL} increase by the same amount, the increase in P_{ALV} must exceed the rise in $P_{LA_{IM}}$, and capillary transmural pressure falls. This increases the volume of Zones 1 and 2 and raises the resistance of the alveolar vessels. At the same time, the increase in elastic recoil that accompanies lung inflation augments the outward traction on the extra-alveolar vessels, which reduces their resistance. This means that the relationship between lung

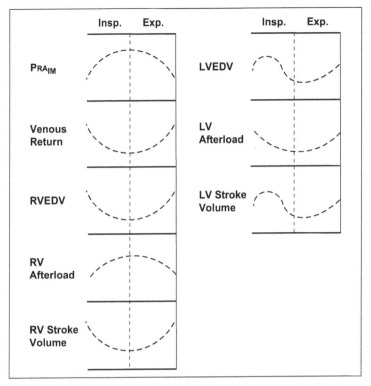

Figure 3.16 Schematic representation of the hemodynamic changes that occur during mechanical ventilation. Insp = inspiration; Exp = expiration

volume and total PVR (and RV afterload) is the same during spontaneous and mechanical ventilation (Figure 3.12).

The Effect on LV Afterload

The rise in P_{PL} during inspiration increases LV end-diastolic pressure. This reduces the amount of pressure that the ventricle must generate to pump blood against the mean arterial pressure, and LV afterload falls. Afterload rises during expiration as P_{PL} returns to baseline.

Factors Affecting the Magnitude of Hemodynamic Changes

The hemodynamic impact of a mechanical breath depends on:

* The level and magnitude of the increase in P_{PL}
* The level and magnitude of the rise in $P_{L_{TM}}$
* Baseline ventricular function

Pleural Pressure

During a mechanical breath, the increase in P_{PL} varies directly with lung volume (Figure 3.17A) and inversely with *chest wall* compliance (Figure 3.17B). This means that, for a given tidal volume, there will be a larger rise in P_{PL} when the chest wall is stiff (e.g., obesity, kyphoscoliosis). Also note that the actual level of P_{PL} becomes much higher as tidal volume increases and chest wall compliance falls. Remember that venous return falls sharply as P_{PL} (and PRA_{IM}) increase and stops completely once PRA_{IM} reaches mean systemic pressure (Figure 3.5).

Lung Transmural Pressure

Figures 3.17A and C show that the increase in PL_{TM} during a mechanical breath is also directly related to tidal volume but inversely related to *lung* compliance. This makes sense if you remember that PL_{TM} is the pressure needed to inflate the lungs. Remember that PVR and RV afterload increase with PL_{TM}.

Ventricular Function

Like during spontaneous breathing, the degree to which changes in venous return alter LV stroke volume and systemic blood pressure depends primarily on baseline LV preload (Figure 3.18). If preload is high, a decrease in LV end-diastolic volume will have little effect on stroke volume. If, however, LV preload is low, any further decrease will cause a significant fall in stroke volume and blood pressure.

This leads to a characteristic, cyclical change in blood pressure. As shown in Figure 3.19, the transient rise in LV preload and stroke volume in early inspiration increases blood pressure. From mid-inspiration to early expiration, blood pressure falls with the drop in LV preload and stroke volume. Between mid-expiration and early inspiration, blood pressure rises with the increase in LV preload.

In patients with preexisting elevated RV afterload or reduced contractility, a marked increase in PL_{TM} may precipitate acute or acute-on-chronic RV failure.

Patient Effort During Mechanical Ventilation

So far, we've only discussed the changes that occur during passive mechanical ventilation. What happens when patients actively inhale and exhale? By directly expanding the chest wall, inspiratory effort reduces the expected increase in P_{PL}, P_{ALV}, and P_{AW}. In fact, vigorous efforts may actually lower these pressures throughout most of inspiration. During active expiration, contraction of the abdominal musculature forces the chest wall down against the lungs, thereby increasing P_{PL} and P_{ALV}. It should be evident, then, that patient effort can significantly change the usual hemodynamic effects of mechanical ventilation.

Positive End-Expiratory Pressure

Positive end-expiratory pressure may be set by the clinician (extrinsic PEEP; $PEEP_E$) or result from dynamic hyperinflation (intrinsic PEEP; $PEEP_I$). The sum of extrinsic and intrinsic PEEP is called *total PEEP* ($PEEP_T$).

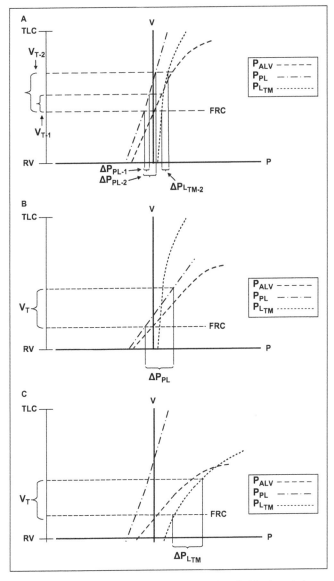

Figure 3.17 (A) Volume–pressure curves illustrating the effect of tidal volume during a mechanical breath. A large tidal volume (V_{T-2}) produces a larger increase and a higher level of pleural pressure (ΔP_{PL-2}) and lung transmural pressure (ΔP_{LTM-2}) than a small tidal volume (V_{T-1}). (B) When chest wall compliance is low, the same tidal volume shown in (A) produces a much larger increase and a much higher level of pleural pressure (ΔP_{PL}). (C) When lung compliance is low, the same tidal volume shown in (A) produces a much larger increase and a much higher level of lung transmural pressure (ΔP_{LTM}).

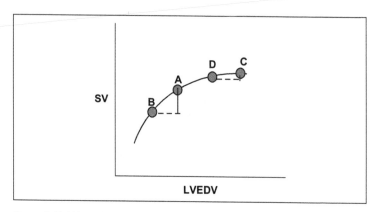

Figure 3.18 When left ventricular end-diastolic volume (LVEDV) and stroke volume (SV) occupy a point on the ascending portion of the ventricular function curve, the decrease in LV preload produced by a mechanical breath (*dashed line*) will cause a relatively large drop in SV (A → B). When ventricular preload is high, the fall in LVEDV has little effect on SV (C → D).

By itself, mechanical ventilation causes only *intermittent* increases in P_{PL} and $P_{L_{TM}}$. As shown in Figure 3.20, PEEP not only augments these pressures during inspiration but *continuously* elevates them throughout the respiratory cycle. This magnifies the hemodynamic effects of mechanical ventilation in proportion to $PEEP_T$. Based on the previous discussion and Figure 3.17, you can see that, for a given level of $PEEP_T$, low *chest wall* compliance will accentuate the rise in P_{PL} and the fall in RV preload, whereas low *lung* compliance will augment the increase in $P_{L_{TM}}$ and RV afterload. Figures 3.17 and 3.20 are extremely important when considering the hemodynamic effects of mechanical ventilation and PEEP in different disease states. You will see them again in later chapters.

The effect of compliance on the rise in P_{PL} and $P_{L_{TM}}$ produced by tidal inflation and PEEP can also be demonstrated mathematically. Recall that the

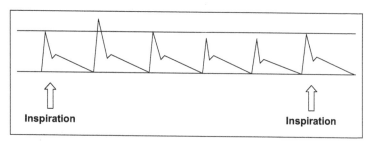

Figure 3.19 The variation in arterial blood pressure during mechanical ventilation in the presence of low LV preload.

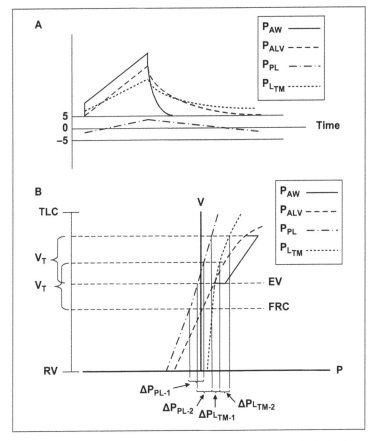

Figure 3.20 (A) Pressure–time curves showing that PEEP elevates airway (P_{AW}), alveolar (P_{ALV}), pleural (P_{PL}), and lung transmural ($P_{L_{TM}}$) pressure throughout the respiratory cycle. (B) Volume–pressure curves showing that PEEP sets a new, higher equilibrium volume (EV) for the respiratory system. The same tidal volume (V_T) produces a similar increase in pleural pressure ($\Delta P_{PL-1} \cong \Delta P_{PL-2}$) and lung transmural pressure ($\Delta P_{L_{TM-1}} \cong \Delta P_{L_{TM-2}}$) with or without PEEP, but the actual values of these pressures are much higher after the addition of PEEP.

compliance of the lungs (C_L) and chest wall (C_{CW}) equals the change in volume (ΔV_L and ΔV_{CW}) divided by the accompanying change in transmural pressure. If we do a little algebra:

$$C_L = \Delta V_L / \Delta \left(P_{ALV} - P_{PL}\right) \quad \text{and} \quad \Delta V_L = C_L \times \Delta \left(P_{ALV} - P_{PL}\right)$$
$$C_{CW} = \Delta V_{CW} / \Delta P_{PL} \quad \text{and} \quad \Delta V_{CW} = C_{CW} \times \Delta P_{PL}$$

Since ΔV_L must equal ΔV_{CW},

$$C_{CW} \times \Delta P_{PL} = C_L \times \Delta(P_{ALV} - P_{PL})$$
$$C_{CW} \times \Delta P_{PL} = (C_L \times \Delta P_{ALV}) - (C_L \times \Delta P_{PL})$$
$$(C_L \times \Delta P_{PL}) + (C_{CW} \times \Delta P_{PL}) = (C_L \times \Delta P_{ALV})$$
$$\Delta P_{PL} \times (C_L + C_{CW}) = (C_L \times \Delta P_{ALV})$$

$$\Delta P_{PL} = \Delta P_{ALV} \times C_L / (C_L + C_{CW}) \qquad (3.9)$$

Let's say that we increase PEEP from 0 to 10 cmH$_2$O. This increases end-expiratory alveolar pressure from 0 to 10 cmH$_2$O, so $\Delta P_{ALV} = 10$ cmH$_2$O. If chest wall compliance is very low (let's say $C_{CW} = 0.1 \times C_L$), Equation 3.9 tells us that P_{PL} increases by 9 cmH$_2$O, but $P_{L_{TM}}$ only increases by $10 - 9 = 1$ cmH$_2$O. If, on the other hand, lung compliance is very low and $C_L = 0.1 \times C_{CW}$, P_{PL} increases by only 0.9 cmH$_2$O, but $P_{L_{TM}}$ goes up by 9.1 cmH$_2$O.

It's usually assumed that venous return falls because of the PEEP-induced increase in P_{PL} and Pra_{IM}; but it's almost certainly not that simple. Several groups of investigators have shown that PEEP reduces venous return despite an *equal increase* in Pra_{IM} and mean systemic pressure. In the absence of a change in driving pressure, it was reasoned and subsequently proven in an animal preparation that PEEP reduces venous return by increasing venous resistance. As shown in Figure 3.5, this reduces the maximal venous return and decreases the slope of the descending portion of the curve.

Mechanical Ventilation and the Cardiovascular System: Take-Home Points

- Mechanical ventilation causes a cyclical increase in P_{PL} and $P_{L_{TM}}$. The increase in P_{PL} (and Pra_{IM}) reduces venous return, RV and LV preload, and LV afterload. The rise in $P_{L_{TM}}$ increases PVR and RV afterload.
- Extrinsic and intrinsic PEEP produce a continuous elevation of P_{PL} and $P_{L_{TM}}$, which further reduces venous return, RV and LV preload, and LV afterload, while increasing RV afterload.
- The hemodynamic significance of these effects depends on the magnitude of the change in P_{PL} and $P_{L_{TM}}$, the actual values of these pressures, and baseline ventricular function:
  - The level of P_{PL} and the magnitude of its increase vary directly with tidal volume and the level of total PEEP and inversely with *chest wall* compliance.
  - The level of $P_{L_{TM}}$ and the magnitude of its increase vary directly with tidal volume and the level of total PEEP and inversely with *lung* compliance.
  - The hemodynamic effect of a given rise in P_{PL} will be greater in patients with low baseline LV preload.
  - The hemodynamic effect of a given rise in $P_{L_{TM}}$ will be greater in patients with baseline RV dysfunction.

Additional Reading

Fessler HE. Heart–lung interactions: Applications in the critically ill. *Eur Respir J.* 1997; 10:226–237.

Feihl F, Broccard AF. Interactions between respiration and systemic hemodynamics. Part I: Basic concepts. *Intensive Care Med.* 2009;35:45–54.

Feihl F, Broccard AF. Interactions between respiration and systemic hemodynamics. Part II: Practical implications in critical care. *Intensive Care Med.* 2009;35:198–205.

Section 2

The Mechanical Ventilator

Congratulations! You made it through my tutorial on essential pulmonary and cardiovascular physiology. It wasn't too bad, was it? Well, even if you had to drink a few grande caramel lattes (with low-fat milk), I guarantee that your newfound knowledge will make it much easier to understand the concepts presented in subsequent chapters. In fact, throughout the rest of this book, I'll often refer to the physiological principles discussed in the previous section, so feel free to go back and reread parts of it as needed. You can always have another latte!

In this next section, you'll learn all about mechanical ventilators, the many options that are available for assisting patient ventilation, and the ventilator alarms that ensure patient safety. You will also become familiar with the huge number of often-confusing abbreviations and acronyms that are used when caring for mechanically ventilated patients.

Chapter 4

Instrumentation and Terminology

General Design

Despite big differences in outward appearance, all mechanical ventilators have several basic features in common (Figure 4.1). All must be connected to *high-pressure sources of oxygen and air*. Once these gases enter the ventilator, they are blended to produce a clinician-selected *fractional inspired oxygen concentration* (F_IO_2). At the onset of inspiration, the *demand valve* opens to allow this pressurized gas to flow through a *heater* and *humidifier*, through the *inspiratory limb* of the ventilator circuit, through the endotracheal tube, and into the patient's lungs. Inspiration ends when the demand valve closes and the *expiratory valve* opens. Exhaled gas travels back to the ventilator through the *expiratory limb* of the ventilator circuit and passes through a *filter* before being released into the atmosphere. Volume and flow are measured each time gas leaves and returns to the ventilator. Airway pressure (P_{AW}) is continuously measured within the ventilator circuit.

All ventilators have a *user interface*, which includes a prominent video display. An example is shown in Figure 4.2.

The user interface serves two important functions. It allows the clinician to easily choose from a wide variety of *ventilator settings* (Box 4.1), and it displays these settings, as well as important, real-time *patient data* (Box 4.2).

Terminology

Boxes 4.1 and 4.2 list most of the terms that you'll need to use and understand when caring for mechanically ventilated patients. So this is a perfect time to tackle ventilator terminology. A few are self-explanatory, but the rest will be reviewed here. Don't worry if you can't remember all of these terms. This is just an introduction. You'll hear much more about these terms (and others will be introduced) in later chapters.

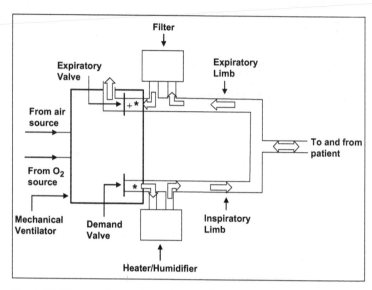

Figure 4.1 Schematic diagram of the ventilator and the ventilator circuit.

* Indicates site of flow and volume measurement

\+ Indicates site of airway pressure measurement

Ventilator Settings (Box 4.1)

The mode of ventilation is the most basic setting because it determines how the patient interacts with the ventilator. In this book, I classify the ventilator modes as:

- Continuous mandatory ventilation (CMV)
- Synchronized intermittent mandatory ventilation (SIMV)
- Spontaneous ventilation (SV)
- Bi-level ventilation

Breath types are defined by their pressure, volume, and flow characteristics, by the signal that ends inspiration, and by the mode(s) with which they can be used. I divide mechanical breaths into five types:

- Volume control (VC)
- Pressure control (PC)
- Adaptive pressure control (aPC)
- Pressure support (PS)
- Adaptive pressure support (aPS)

Chapter 5 is devoted entirely to ventilator modes and breath types.

As discussed in earlier chapters, *positive end-expiratory pressure* (PEEP) is the pressure (in cmH_2O) that remains in the ventilator circuit, airways, and alveoli between mechanical breaths. PEEP increases end-expiratory lung volume

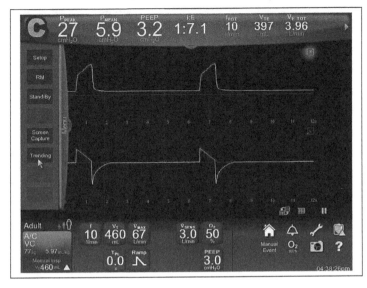

Figure 4.2 A representative ventilator–user interface.

and can improve oxygenation by preventing the collapse of alveoli that were "recruited" during inspiration.

Continuous positive airway pressure (CPAP) is a confusing term because its meaning changes depending on whether it's used during invasive or

---

Box 4.1 Ventilator Settings Available on the User Interface

- Mode
- Breath type
- F_IO_2
- Positive end-expiratory pressure (PEEP)
- Continuous positive airway pressure (CPAP)
- Trigger signal
- Trigger sensitivity
- Mandatory breath rate
- Tidal volume
- Peak inspiratory flow rate
- Flow profile
- Driving pressure
- Inspiratory time
- Plateau time
- Alarms

Box 4.2 Patient Data Displayed on the User Interface

- Graphical displays of pressure, volume, and flow
- Total breath rate
- Mandatory breath rate
- Inspired tidal volume
- Exhaled tidal volume
- Exhaled minute ventilation
- Inspiratory time
- Expiratory time
- Ratio of inspiratory to expiratory time
- Peak airway pressure
- Mean airway pressure
- End-inspiratory (plateau) pressure
- End-expiratory pressure

non-invasive mechanical ventilation (Chapter 16). Just remember that in intubated patients, CPAP has exactly the same meaning as PEEP. That is, it's the amount of pressure maintained in the airways and alveoli throughout expiration. So why do we use this term at all? Well, that's a long story. But, suffice it to say that "CPAP" is sometimes used instead of "PEEP" in the spontaneous ventilation mode (see Chapter 5).

Triggering means that a signal has initiated inspiration by opening the demand valve and closing the expiratory valve. Mechanical breaths are triggered either by the patient (patient-triggered breaths) or, in the absence of sufficient inspiratory effort, by the ventilator (ventilator-triggered breaths).

Most ventilators allow the clinician to choose between two *triggering signals* that indicate patient inspiratory effort. When set to *pressure-triggering*, the demand valve opens once patient effort has lowered the measured airway pressure by a small, clinician-selected amount referred to as the *pressure sensitivity*. For example, as shown in Figure 4.3, if the trigger sensitivity is set at -2 cmH$_2$O and expiratory P$_{AW}$ is zero (atmospheric pressure), a mechanical breath will be triggered whenever patient effort lowers P$_{AW}$ below -2 cmH$_2$O. If P$_{AW}$ is 5 cmH$_2$O during expiration (PEEP), triggering will occur when P$_{AW}$ drops below 3 cmH$_2$O.

Figure 4.4 shows that when *flow-triggering* is used, gas continuously flows at a low rate (the base flow) through the ventilator circuit. When the patient inhales, some of this gas is diverted into the lungs, and the measured expiratory flow falls. A mechanical breath is triggered when the difference between measured inspiratory and expiratory flow exceeds the clinician-selected *flow sensitivity*. For instance, if the base flow is 3 liters per minute (L/min) and the sensitivity is set at 1 L/min, a breath will be triggered every time measured expiratory flow falls below 2 L/min.

Mandatory breaths are delivered by the ventilator with or without patient inspiratory effort, so they are also referred to as "guaranteed"

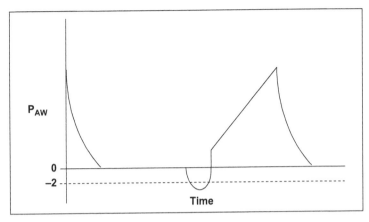

Figure 4.3 Airway pressure (P_{AW}) versus time during a mechanical breath. When set to pressure triggering, the demand valve opens when patient inspiratory effort lowers P_{AW} by the set pressure sensitivity. In this example, expiratory pressure is zero (atmospheric pressure) and sensitivity is set at -2 cmH$_2$O. A breath is triggered when P_{AW} falls below -2 cmH$_2$O.

or "back-up" breaths. *Cycling* refers to the transition between inspiration and expiration, when the demand valve closes and the expiratory valve opens. *Spontaneous breaths* are patient-triggered breaths in excess of the set (mandatory) rate.

When patients receive volume control breaths, some ventilators require the selection of a maximum or *peak inspiratory flow rate* and a *flow profile*, which specifies how the flow rate changes during inspiration. The two common flow profiles are *square-wave*, in which the set peak flow is maintained throughout inspiration, and *descending-ramp*, in which the peak flow occurs early and then steadily falls throughout inspiration (see Chapter 1, Figure 1.11). Other ventilators allow only square-wave flow, which is determined by setting both the tidal volume and the inspiratory time.

The *driving pressure* is a constant, clinician-set pressure that is applied by the ventilator when patients are receiving pressure control and pressure support breaths.

The *inspiratory time* (T_I) is simply the duration of inspiration. It is the interval between triggering and cycling.

Normally, the expiratory valve opens as soon as the demand valve closes and the ventilator then cycles from inspiration to expiration. Clinicians have the option of delaying the opening of the expiratory valve and holding the delivered volume in the lungs by specifying a *plateau time* (see Chapter 1, Figure 1.7).

Ventilator alarms are meant to notify health care providers about a potentially dangerous patient condition or machine malfunction. They've become

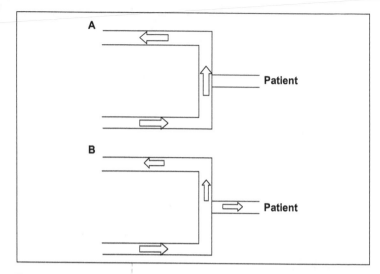

Figure 4.4 (A) Gas flows continuously through the ventilator circuit (the base flow). Since no gas enters the patient's lungs, the flow leaving (inspiratory flow) and returning to the ventilator (expiratory flow) are the same.

(B) When the patient makes an inspiratory effort, some of the base flow is diverted into the lungs. The demand valve opens and a mechanical breath is provided when expiratory flow and inspiratory flow differ by more than the set flow sensitivity.

a very common and, unfortunately, often-ignored sound in most intensive care units (ICUs). Although alarm parameters are typically set by respiratory therapists, it's essential that physicians understand their meaning and potential implications (Table 4.1). Ventilator alarms are discussed in Chapter 6.

Patient Data (Box 4.2)

All ICU ventilators are capable of showing *graphical displays* of real-time patient data. The most commonly used are:

• Airway pressure vs. time
• Flow vs. time
• Flow vs. volume
• Volume vs. airway pressure

The user interface shows the *set* (mandatory) *breath rate*, the *spontaneous breath rate*, and their sum, the *total breath rate*. The *inspired* (delivered) and *exhaled tidal volumes* are also displayed and are normally, of course, very

Table 4.1 Important Ventilator Alarms

Alarm	Common causes	Implications
High airway pressure	Coughing Patient–ventilator asynchrony ET tube or large airway obstruction Pneumothorax	When the high P_{AW} limit is exceeded, the expiratory valve opens, and the patient receives NO VENTILATION.
Low airway pressure	Leak in ventilator circuit Vigorous inspiratory effort	Low tidal volume or excessive work of breathing.
High respiratory rate	Respiratory distress Agitation High ventilation requirements	High patient work of breathing. The patient may need more ventilator support.
Low respiratory rate	Impaired respiratory drive or effort	Ventilation is probably inadequate.
Low exhaled tidal volume	Impaired respiratory drive or effort Leak in ventilator circuit High P_{AW} limit has been exceeded	Ventilation is probably inadequate.

P_{AW} = airway pressure; ET = endotracheal

similar. An isolated drop in exhaled volume usually results either from a leak in the ventilator circuit or from incomplete exhalation. *Inspired and exhaled minute ventilation* are the product of the total breath rate and inspired and exhaled tidal volume, respectively.

Most ventilators also show inspiratory time, *expiratory time* (T_E), and the *ratio of inspiratory to expiratory time* (I:E ratio). The expiratory time is the interval between mechanical breaths, so it's also the maximum time that the patient has to exhale the delivered tidal volume. It's determined by T_I and the total breath rate. For example, if a patient breathes at a rate of 20 times per minute, the average respiratory cycle length is 60/20, or 3 seconds. If T_I is 1 second, then T_E must be 2 seconds. The *I:E* ratio is normally less than 1.

The *peak airway pressure* (P_{PEAK}) is the maximum pressure reached during the preceding mechanical breath. The *mean airway pressure* (P_{MEAN}) is continuously calculated by averaging airway pressure throughout the entire respiratory cycle (inspiration and expiration).

The *end-inspiratory* or *plateau pressure* (P_{PLAT}) is measured and displayed after a clinician-set delay between closure of the demand valve and opening of the expiratory valve. This can be done on most machines by setting a plateau time (see preceding), or more commonly, by simply initiating a brief pause through the user interface. As discussed in Chapter 1, the plateau pressure is the *total elastic recoil pressure* of the respiratory system at the end of inspiration.

The *end-expiratory pressure* is measured and displayed when the clinician closes the expiratory valve just before the next breath. On all ventilators, this can easily be done via the user interface. This pressure, which is also referred to as total PEEP ($PEEP_T$), is the sum of the set level of PEEP (extrinsic PEEP; $PEEP_E$) and intrinsic PEEP ($PEEP_I$), which results from incomplete exhalation and dynamic hyperinflation.

Chapter 5

Ventilator Modes and Breath Types

Mechanical ventilators allow the clinician to choose among many different ways of providing or assisting patient ventilation. The most important settings are the mode of ventilation and the type of mechanical breath. Although all machines provide very similar, if not identical, options, terminology varies widely among manufacturers (and authors). So it's very difficult to read a review article or a textbook (even this one) and understand what the different settings on *your* ventilator actually do. There have been surprisingly few attempts to standardize ventilator terminology, although Chatburn and colleagues have proposed a "taxonomy" for mechanical ventilation (see "Additional Reading" at the end of this chapter). To give you some idea of the magnitude of this problem, Table 5.1 matches the classification scheme used in this book with the terms used by several ventilator companies and authors.

If you really want to understand the ventilator(s) used in your hospital, my advice is to make a trip to the respiratory therapy department and borrow (and read) the manufacturer's user manual. I'm not kidding! The relevant sections are fairly short, and it will allow you to understand how your particular machine works and the terminology it uses.

As mentioned in Chapter 4, the *mode of ventilation* is the most basic ventilator setting and can be thought of simply as defining how the ventilator and the patient interact. It is usually the first parameter chosen by the clinician and influences many subsequent settings. The *type of mechanical breath* determines how the ventilator provides the pressure, volume, and flow needed to inflate the lungs. As you can see from Table 5.1, the mode and breath type are usually combined to form a complex abbreviation, such as CMV-VC and SPONT-PS.

Modes of Mechanical Ventilation

Continuous Mandatory Ventilation (CMV)

The CMV mode is also commonly referred to as *assist-control (AC) ventilation*. The CMV mode provides the patient with a clinician-selected number of guaranteed mechanical breaths each minute. These *mandatory breaths* can be triggered in two ways. The patient can initiate a breath simply by making an adequate inspiratory effort (patient-triggered breaths), or, in the absence of

Table 5.1 Comparison of Terms and Abbreviations Used for Ventilator Modes and Breath Types

My classification	Medtronic (Puritan-Bennett)	Maquet	Drager	Hamilton	Other terms
CMV-VC	A/C-VC	VC	VC-AC	CMV	Volume A/C
CMV-PC	A/C-PC	PC	PC-AC	P-CMV	Pressure A/C
CMV-aPC	A/C-VC+	PRVC	PC-AC-VG	APVcmv	VTPC, VAPC
SIMV-VC	SIMV-VC	SIMV (VC) + PS	VC-SIMV	SIMV	
SIMV-PC	SIMV-PC	SIMV (PC) + PS	PC-SIMV	P-SIMV	
SIMV-aPC	SIMV-VC+	SIMV (PRVC) + PS	PC-SIMV-VG	APVsimv	
SPONT-PS	SPONT-PS	PS	SPN-CPAP/PS	SPONT	
SPONT-aPS	SPONT-VS	VS	SPN-CPAP/VS	VS	
Bi-Level	Bi-Level	Bi-Vent	PC-BiPap PC-APRV	DuoPAP APRV	

CMV = Continuous Mandatory Ventilation; SIMV = Synchronized Intermittent Mandatory Ventilation; SPONT and SPN = Spontaneous Ventilation; VC = Volume Control; PC and P = Pressure Control; aPC = Adaptive Pressure Control; aPS = Adaptive Pressure Support; A/C and AC = Assist-Control; VS = Volume Support; PRVC = Pressure-Regulated Volume Control; VG = Volume Guarantee; CPAP = Continuous Positive Airway Pressure; APRV = Airway Pressure Release Ventilation; APV = Adaptive Pressure Ventilation; VTPC = Volume-Targeted Pressure Control; VAPC = Volume-Assured Pressure Control

patient effort, the ventilator will deliver a mandatory breath at regular intervals (ventilator-triggered breaths).

These two triggering methods are shown in Figure 5.1. Note that the ventilator uses the set (mandatory) rate to divide each minute into equal breath intervals. For example, if the rate is set at 10 per minute, each interval is 60 seconds ÷ 10, or 6 seconds. In the absence of patient effort, a ventilator-triggered breath is provided at the end of each interval (Figure 5.1A). During active inspiration, however (Figure 5.1B), a mandatory breath is triggered by the first patient effort of each interval, and a ventilator-triggered breath is given only if the patient is apneic for an entire cycle.

Although the patient is guaranteed to receive a set number of mandatory breaths, the CMV mode allows any number of additional patient-triggered breaths, as shown in Figure 5.1C. Note that within each breath interval, these *spontaneous breaths* always follow a mandatory breath and that mandatory and spontaneous breaths are identical.

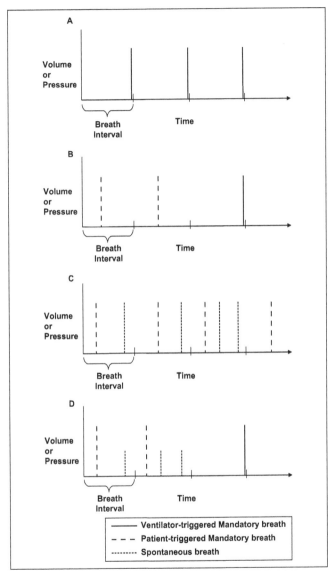

Figure 5.1 In the CMV and SIMV modes, if the patient is apneic (A), all mandatory breaths are ventilator-triggered and occur at the end of each calculated breath interval. If the patient breathes at or below the set rate (B), some mandatory breaths will be patient-triggered, while others will be ventilator-triggered. If the patient's respiratory rate exceeds the set rate (C, D), all mandatory and spontaneous breaths will be triggered by the patient. In the CMV mode (C), spontaneous and mandatory breaths are identical. In the SIMV mode (D), they are always different.

The CMV mode may be used with volume control (VC), pressure control (PC), and adaptive pressure control (aPC) breaths.

A summary of the CMV mode is provided in Box 5.1.

Box 5.1 Summary of the CMV Mode

Features

- Clinician-set mandatory breath rate
- Mandatory breaths may be patient-triggered or ventilator-triggered
- The patient may trigger any number of additional (spontaneous) breaths
- Mandatory and spontaneous breaths are identical

Clinician-Set Parameters

- Mandatory breath rate
- Breath type
  - VC
  - PC
  - aPC
- Fractional inspired O_2 concentration (F_IO_2)
- Positive end-expiratory pressure (PEEP)

Synchronized Intermittent Mandatory Ventilation (SIMV)

The SIMV mode is very similar to the CMV mode. In fact, if the patient is apneic or breathes at or below the set mandatory rate, the two modes are identical (Figure 5.1A and 5.1B). Like CMV, SIMV provides the patient with a clinician-selected mandatory breath rate, and a single mandatory breath, which can be either ventilator- or patient-triggered, is provided during each calculated breath interval. The difference between the two modes only appears when the patient triggers additional spontaneous breaths. In the CMV mode, spontaneous and mandatory breaths are the same; but in the SIMV mode, different breath types are always used (Figure 5.1D). Like CMV, mandatory breaths in the SIMV mode can be VC, PC, or aPC breaths. Spontaneous breaths, however, must be pressure support (PS) breaths. The SIMV mode is summarized in Box 5.2.

Spontaneous Ventilation

The spontaneous mode provides no mandatory breaths. All mechanical breaths must be spontaneous and triggered by the patient (Figure 5.2). The spontaneous mode can be used only with PS or adaptive pressure support (aPS) breaths. Box 5.3 provides a summary of this mode.

Bi-level Ventilation

In this mode, patients cycle between a high and low clinician-set level of positive airway pressure (Figure 5.3). What distinguishes this mode from

Box 5.2 Summary of the SIMV Mode

Features

- Clinician-set mandatory breath rate
- Mandatory breaths may be patient-triggered or ventilator-triggered
- The patient may trigger any number of additional (spontaneous) breaths
- Mandatory and spontaneous breaths are always different

Clinician-Set Parameters

- Mandatory breath rate
- Mandatory breath type
  - VC
  - PC
  - aPC
- Spontaneous breath type
  - PS
- F_IO_2
- PEEP

CMV with PC breaths is that patients may trigger spontaneous (pressure support) breaths at both pressure levels. Note that the pressure support level during high-pressure spontaneous breaths is limited to prevent dangerously high inspiratory pressures; as shown in Figure 5.3A, a common approach is to limit inspiratory pressure to the sum of the low pressure level and the set PS level. In the bi-level mode, ventilation occurs during spontaneous breaths and during the transitions between the two pressure

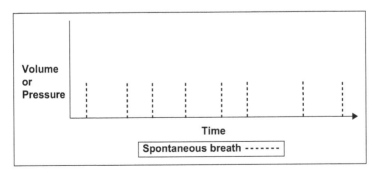

Figure 5.2 In the spontaneous mode, there are no mandatory breaths, and all breaths must be triggered by the patient.

Box 5.3 Summary of the Spontaneous Mode

Features

• No mandatory breaths
• All breaths are spontaneous and patient-triggered

Clinician-Set Parameters

• Breath type
  • PS
  • aPS
• F$_I$O$_2$
• PEEP

levels. Airway pressure release ventilation (APRV) is a variant of this mode in which the low-pressure interval (the pressure release) is very brief, and the ratio of high to low pressure duration is greater than 1.0 (Figure 5.3B). Box 5.4 summarizes the bi-level mode.

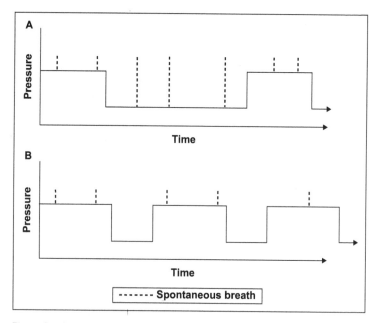

Figure 5.3 (A) In the bi-level mode, airway pressure alternates between high and low clinician-set levels. The patient may trigger spontaneous breaths at both levels.

(B) Airway pressure release ventilation (APRV) is a variant of bi-level ventilation that has only brief periods of low pressure.

Box 5.4 Summary of the Bi-level Mode

Features
- Airway pressure alternates between a high and low set level
- The patient may trigger spontaneous breaths at both levels of airway pressure

Clinician-Set Parameters
- High airway pressure
- Low airway pressure
- Duration of high airway pressure
- Duration of low airway pressure
- Pressure support level
- F_iO_2

Types of Mechanical Breaths

At the most basic level, the breaths available on ICU ventilators can be divided into two types. *Volume-set breaths* provide a clinician-selected tidal volume, whereas *pressure-set breaths* maintain a set, constant airway pressure throughout inspiration. As we will discuss in much greater detail, the pressure needed to deliver a set volume and the volume generated by a specified pressure depend on a number of factors that vary between patients and even in the same patient over time. So, volume-set breaths are *pressure-variable*, and pressure-set breaths are *volume-variable*. Each of the breath types discussed here can also be differentiated by its flow characteristics, by the signal that ends inspiration (*cycling*), and by the mode(s) with which it can be used.

Volume Control (VC)

Volume control breaths provide the patient with a clinician-selected, guaranteed tidal volume. On some ventilators, the maximum (peak) flow rate and flow profile (constant or descending ramp) must also be specified. On these machines, inspiratory time (T_I) is not set, but instead depends on the selected tidal volume (V_T) and the mean flow rate ($\dot{V}_{mean}$), which, in turn, depends on the selected peak flow and flow profile.

$$T_I = V_T / \dot{V}_{mean} \tag{5.1}$$

For example, a VC breath with a set volume of 0.5 L and a constant flow of 1 L/sec will have a T_I of 0.5 second. Other ventilators provide only constant flow that is determined by the clinician-set T_I and V_T.

$$\dot{V} = V_T / T_I \tag{5.2}$$

So, a V_T of 0.5 L with a T_I of 0.5 second will generate a constant flow of 1 L/sec.

Volume control breaths are *time-cycled*. That is, the demand valve closes, inspiratory flow stops, and the expiratory valve opens once the set or calculated (Equation 5.1) inspiratory time has elapsed. Volume control breaths can be used only with the CMV and SIMV modes.

Volume control breaths are *volume-set* and *pressure-variable*, so let's look at what determines how much pressure is needed. I actually spent a long time discussing this in Chapter 1 (see Figures 1.9, 1.11, and 1.14), although there, I didn't specify that I was talking about VC breaths. Recall that the pressure generated by the ventilator (P_{AW}) during a *passive* (i.e., no patient effort) VC breath must always equal the sum of the pressures needed to overcome viscous forces (P_V), the increase in elastic recoil produced by the delivered volume (P_{ER}), and total end-expiratory pressure ($PEEP_T$).

$$P_{AW} = P_V + P_{ER} + PEEP_T \qquad (5.3)$$

Since P_{ER} is equal to the delivered volume (ΔV) divided by the compliance of the respiratory system (C_{RS}), and P_V equals the product of airway resistance (R) and flow ($\dot{V}$), we can rewrite this equation as:

$$P_{AW} = (R \times \dot{V}) + (\Delta V / C) + PEEP_T \qquad (5.4)$$

Figure 5.4 shows plots of P_{AW} and alveolar pressure (P_{ALV}) versus time during passive VC breaths with constant inspiratory flow. As discussed in Chapter 1, P_{ALV} is equal to the sum of P_{ER} and $PEEP_T$, and P_V is the difference between P_{AW} and P_{ALV}. Since flow is constant, volume, elastic recoil, and P_{ALV} increase linearly throughout inspiration. P_{AW} also increases linearly and reaches its peak pressure (P_{PEAK}) at end-inspiration. As predicted by Equation 5.4, both P_{PEAK} and end-inspiratory P_{ALV} increase (with no change in P_V) when tidal volume increases or compliance falls. When resistance or flow rises, P_V and P_{PEAK} increase without changing P_{ALV}. P_{PEAK} and end-inspiratory P_{ALV} also increase when PEEP is present. A decrease in resistance, flow, volume, or $PEEP_T$, and an increase in compliance have the opposite effects. Note that inspiratory time varies with tidal volume and flow, as predicted by Equation 5.1.

Now let's look at Figure 5.5, which shows how and why the shape of the P_{AW} curve changes with the inspiratory flow profile. This was also discussed in Chapter 1. If resistance is constant, P_V varies only with the rate of gas flow. If flow is constant (Figures 5.4 and 5.5A), P_V will also be constant. If a descending ramp pattern of flow is used (Figure 5.5B), P_V progressively falls, P_{ALV} approaches P_{AW}, and P_{PEAK} drops. Also notice that by reducing mean flow, a descending ramp profile increases the time required to deliver the set tidal volume (T_I).

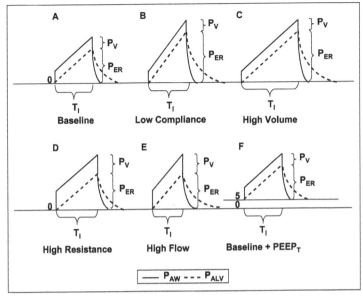

Figure 5.4 Schematic representation of the effect of low compliance (B), high volume (C), high resistance (D), high flow (E), and $PEEP_T$ (F) on baseline (A) airway pressure (P_{AW}) and alveolar pressure (P_{ALV}) during volume control breaths with constant inspiratory flow. The pressure needed to balance elastic recoil (P_{ER}) and overcome viscous forces (P_V) at end-inspiration and inspiratory time (T_I) are shown. When $PEEP_T$ is zero (Figure 5.4A–5.4E), P_{ALV} equals P_{ER}. When PEEP is present (Figure 5.4F), P_{ALV} equals the sum of P_{ER} and $PEEP_T$.

So far, we have considered the factors that determine P_{AW} only during a passive VC breath. When a patient inhales, the pressure produced by the diaphragm and other inspiratory muscles helps overcome elastic recoil and viscous forces. Since inspiratory flow cannot increase, the pressure in the ventilator circuit falls. As shown in Figure 5.6, increasing inspiratory effort causes a progressive change in the shape of the P_{AW}-time curve and may even lower P_{PEAK}.

A summary of volume control breaths is provided in Box 5.5.

Pressure Control (PC)

When delivering PC breaths, the ventilator maintains a constant P_{AW} throughout inspiration. The clinician sets this pressure by selecting the *driving pressure* (DP) that is applied at the onset of inspiration. Inspiratory pressure is then the sum of the DP and the set level of PEEP. Inspiratory time must also be specified. Pressure control breaths are therefore *pressure-set* and *time-cycled*. They can be used only with the CMV and SIMV modes.

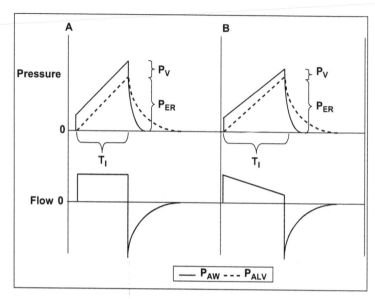

Figure 5.5 On some ventilators, volume control breaths allow the clinician to choose a constant (A) or a descending-ramp (B) flow profile. Peak airway pressure (P_{PEAK}), the pressure needed to overcome viscous forces (P_V), and inspiratory time (T_I) change with the selected flow profile. If tidal volume and compliance are constant, the pressure needed to balance elastic recoil (P_{ER}) does not change.

Figure 5.7 illustrates the differences between the P_{AW}, P_{ALV}, flow, and volume curves of passive VC and PC breaths. Let's see why these differences occur. Remember from Chapter 1 that airway resistance is equal to the gradient between P_{AW} and P_{ALV} divided by flow.

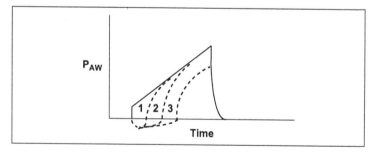

Figure 5.6 The effect of varying levels of patient inspiratory effort on airway pressure (P_{AW}) during a volume control breath. As effort increases (1 → 2 → 3), there is progressive alteration of the P_{AW}–time curve.

Box 5.5 Summary of Volume Control Breaths

Features

• Volume-set
• Pressure-variable
• Set flow or inspiratory time
• Time-cycled
• Used with CMV and SIMV modes

Clinician-Set Parameters

• Tidal volume
• Peak flow and flow profile OR inspiratory time

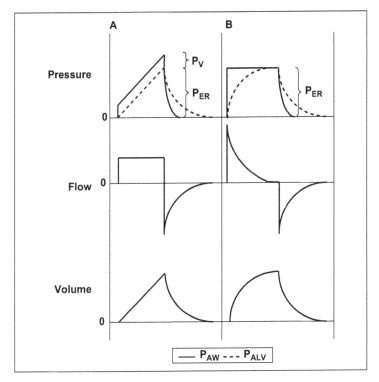

Figure 5.7 Schematic diagram showing the differences in airway pressure (P_{AW}), alveolar pressure (P_{ALV}), flow, and volume during passive volume control (A) and pressure control (B) breaths. Since tidal volume and compliance are the same, the pressure needed to balance elastic recoil (P_{ER}) doesn't change. Because flow stops before the end of inspiration, no pressure is needed to overcome viscous forces (P_V) during the pressure control breath, and this lowers peak airway pressure.

$$R = (P_{AW} - P_{ALV}) / \dot{V} \qquad (5.5)$$

By rearranging this equation, we can calculate the flow at any time ($\dot{V}t$).

$$\dot{V}t = (P_{AW} - P_{ALV}) / R \qquad (5.6)$$

Because P_{AW} is constant, Equation 5.6 tells us that flow is highest at the beginning of inspiration when P_{ALV} is at its lowest level. Flow must then progressively fall as the lungs expand, P_{ALV} rises, and the gradient between P_{AW} and P_{ALV} decreases. Flow will stop when P_{AW} and P_{ALV} become equal. Because of the shape of the flow-time curve and because flow is simply volume per time, lung volume increases much more rapidly than during a VC breath. End-inspiratory P_{ALV} is the same in Figures 5.7A and 5.7B because the delivered volume is the same. But end-inspiratory P_{AW} (P_{PEAK}) is lower during PC breaths because flow (and P_V) is minimal or absent.

Now let's see how PC breaths are affected by changes in driving pressure, resistance, and compliance (Figure 5.8). We'll start by focusing on inspiratory flow. Look again at Equation 5.6. If driving pressure (and P_{AW}) is increased, flow

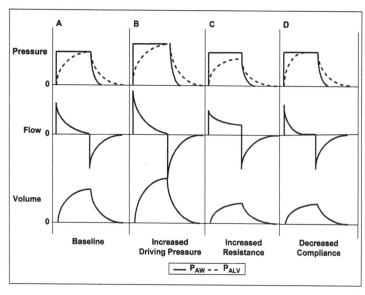

Figure 5.8 Schematic diagram showing how an increase in driving pressure (B) and resistance (C) and a fall in compliance (D) alter baseline (A) airway pressure (P_{AW}), alveolar pressure (P_{ALV}), flow, and volume during pressure control breaths.

must also increase throughout inspiration (Figure 5.8B). When resistance is high, flow must fall (Figure 5.8C), and this means that it takes longer for P_{AW} and P_{ALV} to equilibrate. In fact, flow will persist at end-inspiration unless the set T_I is sufficient to allow P_{ALV} to reach P_{AW}. When compliance is low (Figure 5.8D), P_{ALV} rises quickly to reach P_{AW}, and the duration of inspiratory flow is reduced.

Now let's look at tidal volume. Recall from Chapter 1 that compliance (C) is the ratio of the volume change (ΔV) produced by a change in pressure (ΔP).

$$C = \Delta V / \Delta P \tag{5.7}$$

If we rearrange this equation, you can see that the tidal volume (V_T) delivered by each PC breath is determined by respiratory system compliance and the difference between P_{ALV} at the end of expiration (P_{ALVee}) and the end of inspiration (P_{ALVei}).

$$V_T = \left(P_{ALVei} - P_{ALVee} \right) \times C \tag{5.8}$$

Since P_{ALV} and P_{AW} are usually equal at end-inspiration, Equation 5.8 can also be written as:

$$V_T = \left(P_{AW} - P_{ALVee} \right) \times C \tag{5.9}$$

This means that V_T will increase with DP (Figure 5.8B) and fall with respiratory system compliance (Figure 5.8D). As you can see from Equation 5.8 and Figure 5.8C, V_T will also fall if high resistance prevents P_{AW} and P_{ALV} from equilibrating before the end of inspiration (i.e., $P_{ALVei} < P_{AW}$).

The opposite effects from those shown in Figure 5.8 will occur with a decrease in DP, a fall in airway resistance, and an increase in respiratory system compliance.

During VC breaths, increasing patient effort causes P_{AW} to fall but does not change inspiratory flow or volume (Figure 5.6). During PC breaths, P_{AW} remains constant, but flow and volume vary with patient effort. That's because inspiratory effort lowers P_{ALV} and increases the P_{AW}–P_{ALV} gradient. So, the greater the effort, the more flow and volume the patient will receive. Since PC breaths typically have a short set T_I, though, the patient has relatively little time to influence flow and volume.

Now that you understand the basics of PC breaths, we have to discuss the effect of PEEP (Figure 5.9). Remember from Chapter 1 that $PEEP_T$ is P_{ALV} at end-expiration and the sum of intentionally added or extrinsic PEEP ($PEEP_E$) and intrinsic PEEP ($PEEP_I$). This allows us to rewrite Equation 5.9 as:

$$V_T = \left(P_{AW} - PEEP_T \right) \times C \tag{5.10}$$

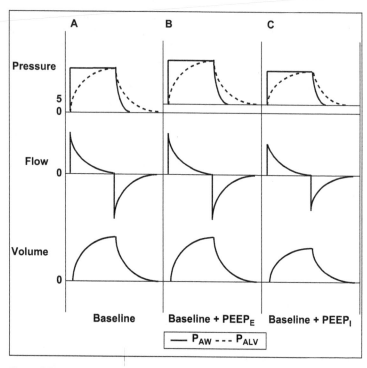

Figure 5.9 Airway (P_{AW}) and alveolar (P_{ALV}) pressure, flow, and volume curves during pressure control breaths with PEEP of 0 (A) extrinsic PEEP ($PEEP_E$) of 5 cmH$_2$O (B) and intrinsic PEEP ($PEEP_I$) of 5 cmH$_2$O (C). Driving pressure, flow, and volume are unchanged by $PEEP_E$ but fall when $PEEP_I$ is present.

Since the ventilator adjusts P_{AW} for $PEEP_E$ (i.e., $P_{AW} = DP + PEEP_E$), the DP, flow, and tidal volume remain unchanged (Figure 5.9B). Unfortunately, the ventilator cannot detect or adjust for $PEEP_I$. So, as $PEEP_I$ and $PEEP_T$ increase, the DP ($P_{AW} - PEEP_T$) and the delivered tidal volume (and flow) fall (Figure 5.9C). So watch out whenever you make a change that decreases expiratory time, such as increasing the mandatory rate or T_I, because it may cause a significant drop in V_T. Pressure-control breaths are summarized in Box 5.6.

Adaptive Pressure Control (aPC)

This breath type, which is also referred to by a variety of other names, including *pressure-regulated volume control (PRVC)*, *volume control plus (VC+)*, *volume-targeted pressure control (VTPC)*, and *volume-assured pressure control (VAPC)*, is a hybrid of VC and PC breaths. In essence, aPC uses a pressure control breath to deliver a clinician-set tidal volume. Since mechanical breaths can be volume-set or pressure-set, but not both, you're probably wondering how this

> ## Box 5.6 Summary of Pressure Control Breaths
>
> ### Features
>
> - Pressure-set
> - Volume-variable
> - Flow-variable
> - Time-cycled
> - Used with CMV and SIMV modes
>
> ### Clinician-Set Parameters
>
> - Driving pressure
> - Inspiratory time

is done. The answer is that, like PC breaths, aPC breaths maintain a constant P_{AW} throughout inspiration, but the ventilator adjusts this pressure to deliver a target tidal volume.

When aPC is selected, the clinician sets both the tidal volume and the inspiratory time. Initially, the ventilator delivers a series of pressure control breaths until it determines the pressure needed to generate the set volume. Exhaled volume is then constantly monitored, and inspiratory airway pressure is adjusted to maintain this volume. If volume falls, P_{AW} is increased; if volume increases, P_{AW} is reduced. Like VC and PC breaths, aPC breaths can be used only with the CMV and SIMV modes.

You can see that aPC breaths overcome the major drawback of PC breaths—the marked change in delivered tidal volume (and minute ventilation) that can occur due to changes in compliance, resistance, patient effort, and $PEEP_I$. Adaptive pressure control breaths compensate for these factors by adjusting P_{AW}, thereby eliminating the volume variability inherent in PC breaths. Box 5.7 provides a summary of aPC breaths.

> ## Box 5.7 Summary of aPC Breaths
>
> ### Features
>
> - Volume-set
> - Pressure-variable (between patients and between breaths)
> - Flow-variable
> - Time-cycled
> - Used with CMV and SIMV modes
>
> ### Clinician-Set Parameters
>
> - Tidal volume
> - Inspiratory time

Pressure Support (PS)

Like PC breaths, PS breaths provide a constant airway pressure that is the sum of a clinician-selected driving pressure (now called the *pressure support level*) and PEEP$_E$. Unlike PC breaths, however, inspiratory time is not set. Instead, the ventilator cycles only when inspiratory flow falls below a low, preset value. So PS breaths are *pressure-set* and *flow-cycled*. Pressure support breaths are used in the SIMV, spontaneous ventilation, and bi-level modes.

Since PS breaths are pressure-set, inspiratory flow and tidal volume are influenced by the set pressure, respiratory system compliance and resistance, and PEEP$_I$, just as they are with PC breaths; and, like PC breaths, inspiratory effort during PS breaths lowers P$_{ALV}$ and increases the P$_{AW}$–P$_{ALV}$ gradient, which allows patients to influence inspiratory flow rate and tidal volume.

The big (actually huge) difference between these two breath types results from how they are cycled. Since inspiratory flow doesn't stop until some minimum value has been reached, PS breaths give the patient total control over

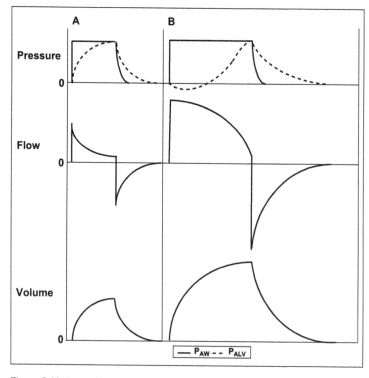

Figure 5.10 Airway (P$_{AW}$) and alveolar (P$_{ALV}$) pressure, flow, and volume curves during pressure support breaths with minimal (A) and large (B) patient inspiratory effort. Flow, volume, and inspiratory time increase with patient effort.

Box 5.8 Summary of Pressure Support Breaths

Features

- Pressure-set
- Volume-variable
- Flow-variable
- Flow-cycled
- Used with SIMV, spontaneous ventilation, and bi-level modes

Clinician-Set Parameters

- Pressure support level

---

inspiratory time. So, for example, if the patient generates only the minimal effort needed to trigger the ventilator, T_I will be short, and inspiratory flow and tidal volume will be determined only by the set PS level and respiratory system compliance and resistance. If, on the other hand, the patient puts a lot of effort into breathing, inspiration will not end until the patient stops inhaling, and inspiratory flow and volume will be much greater. The effect of patient effort on T_I, flow, and volume is shown in Figure 5.10. Box 5.8 summarizes pressure support breaths.

Adaptive Pressure Support (aPS)

Adaptive pressure support breaths, which are most commonly referred to as *volume support* breaths, are similar to aPC breaths because they deliver a clinician-set tidal volume while maintaining a constant P_{AW}. Also, like aPC breaths, exhaled tidal volume is monitored, and P_{AW} is adjusted to maintain the set volume. The difference is that aPS breaths use a pressure support rather than a pressure control breath. Adaptive pressure support breaths eliminate the potentially marked volume variability of PS breaths by altering P_{AW} to compensate for changes in compliance, resistance, $PEEP_I$, and, most importantly, patient effort. Adaptive pressure support breaths can be used only with the spontaneous ventilation mode. Box 5.9 provides a summary.

Box 5.9 Summary of Adaptive Pressure Support Breaths

Features

- Volume-set
- Pressure-variable (between patients and between breaths)
- Flow-variable
- Flow-cycled
- Used with spontaneous ventilation mode

Clinician-Set Parameters

- Tidal volume

How and When to Use Ventilator Modes and Breath Types

How do you decide which mode and breath type to use for a particular patient? Well, I'm going to make this simple—because it is.

The course of patients who require mechanical ventilation can be divided into two phases. In the first, which I'll call the *critical illness phase*, the patient requires lots of support from the ventilator. If the patient survives, they usually improve to the point that mechanical ventilation may no longer be needed. I'll call this the *recovery phase*.

For patients in the critical illness phase, CMV is by far the most commonly used mode of mechanical ventilation, and there are several good reasons for this. First, CMV provides a mandatory respiratory rate, so it can be set to guarantee a minimum, safe minute ventilation (and $PaCO_2$ and pH). Second, by allowing additional spontaneous breaths, CMV lets the patient set the amount of ventilation needed for optimum CO_2 clearance. Finally, CMV significantly reduces patient effort and work of breathing, because all mechanical breaths, whether mandatory or spontaneous, provide the same tidal volume and can be triggered by a minimal amount of inspiratory effort. This is obviously important in patients who are unable to maintain adequate spontaneous ventilation.

The other modes are simply less appropriate. Spontaneous ventilation isn't safe because it doesn't provide mandatory breaths. SIMV is also problematic because adequate minute ventilation depends on the patient's ability to generate sufficient volume with each spontaneous breath. This, of course, also increases patient work of breathing. Bi-level ventilation has the same drawbacks as SIMV because it also uses PS breaths. It is occasionally used to improve PaO_2 by opening or "recruiting" atelectatic alveoli in patients with ARDS (see Chapter 12), but there's no evidence that it has a role in the routine management of these patients.

Once you've selected the CMV mode, you have three breath types to choose from: VC, PC, and aPC. If you think about it, VC breaths are ideal for critically ill patients because they provide a set tidal volume. This is essential for patients whose inspiratory effort, compliance, and resistance are likely to change repeatedly and unpredictably. Adaptive pressure control breaths are also acceptable, because they, too, are volume-set. Some clinicians favor aPC breaths because they believe that allowing some control over inspiratory flow improves patient comfort. Since P_{ALV} rises faster and mean P_{ALV} is higher than during VC breaths (Figure 5.7), aPC breaths may also increase alveolar recruitment and improve PaO_2, and are sometimes preferentially used in patients with ARDS. Because they are volume-variable, PC breaths must be used with caution in critically ill patients.

What about patients who have entered the recovery phase of their illness? As I will discuss in Chapter 15, "spontaneous breathing trials" are used to determine whether mechanical ventilation can be discontinued. These can be truly spontaneous with no ventilator assistance (i.e., a "T-piece"), or the patient can be switched from CMV to spontaneous ventilation with a small amount (e.g., 5 cmH$_2$O) of pressure support. I prefer the latter because it's less time-consuming for the respiratory therapist, and all ventilator alarms remain active. Either way, the patient is considered for extubation if they demonstrate adequate spontaneous ventilation for 30 to 60 minutes. Patients who do poorly during a spontaneous breathing trial are returned to the CMV mode.

So, in the spirit of keeping it simple, here are my recommendations:

- Use CMV-VC or CMV-aPC in critically ill patients with respiratory failure.
- Assess the patient's ability to breathe spontaneously by changing from CMV to spontaneous ventilation and adding a low level of pressure support.

Additional Reading

Blanch PB, Jones M, Layon AJ, Camner N. Pressure-preset ventilation. Part 1: physiologic and mechanical considerations. *Chest*. 1993;104:590–599.

Blanch PB, Jones M, Layon AJ, Camner N. Pressure-preset ventilation. Part 2: mechanics and safety. *Chest*. 1993;104:904–912.

Chatburn RL, El-Khatib M, Mireles-Cabodevila E. A taxonomy for mechanical ventilation: 10 fundamental maxims. *Respir Care*. 2014;59:1747–1763.

Mireles-Cabodevila E, Hatipoglu U, Chatburn RL. A rational framework for selecting modes of ventilation. *Respir Care*. 2013;58:348–366.

Chapter 6

Ventilator Alarms— Causes and Evaluation

When a patient is intubated and placed on mechanical ventilation, the clinician must write a series of ventilator orders, and this will be covered in Chapter 8. It's important to recognize, though, that several other parameters are typically set by the respiratory therapist without direct physician input. The most important are the critical values that will trigger a ventilator alarm.

ICU ventilators constantly monitor many machine and patient-related variables, including airway pressure, flow rate, volume, and respiratory rate, and it seems like there's an alarm for almost everything. Unfortunately, since these alarms are so common, many nurses and physicians either ignore them or reflexively "silence" them through the user interface. While it's true that some alarms are of little or no significance, others may indicate an important and potentially life-threatening problem. That's why it's essential that all physicians caring for mechanically ventilated patients be able to identify the reason for every ventilator alarm and understand its causes and implications. Ventilator alarms are listed in Box 6.1.

Once an alarm sounds, you can determine its meaning and significance only by going to the bedside and looking at the user interface. There, most ventilators display the reason for the current alarm(s)—yes, there can be more than one at a time—and even show which alarms have been active in the recent past. Once you identify the specific alarm, you need to determine its potential causes and know how to quickly and accurately diagnose and correct the problem.

In this chapter, I will discuss only the most common and clinically important ventilator alarms. These are:

- High airway pressure
- Low airway pressure
- High respiratory rate
- Low respiratory rate
- Low exhaled tidal volume

Box 6.1 Ventilator Alarms

- AC power loss
- Apnea
- Circuit disconnect
- High airway pressure
- Low airway pressure
- High exhaled tidal volume
- Low exhaled tidal volume
- High minute ventilation
- Low minute ventilation
- High respiratory rate
- Low respiratory rate
- Low F_iO_2
- High PEEP
- Low PEEP

PEEP = positive end-expiratory pressure; F_iO_2 = fractional inspired O_2 concentration

High Airway Pressure

Recall that the pressure generated by the ventilator (airway pressure; P_{AW}) is constantly measured proximal to the expiratory valve. On most machines, it is displayed both graphically in real-time as a pressure–time curve and digitally as the maximum or peak (P_{PEAK}) airway pressure during the preceding breath. After mechanical ventilation is initiated, the respiratory therapist will set a *high airway pressure limit*, which is typically 15–20 cmH$_2$O above P_{PEAK}.

It's important to understand that when P_{AW} exceeds the set pressure limit, the ventilator immediately cycles from inspiration to expiration, and the patient receives no gas flow. So, until the underlying problem has been identified and corrected, the patient will get very little if any ventilation!

The most common cause of a high airway pressure alarm is the spike in P_{AW} produced when a patient coughs. This is almost always self-limited and requires no intervention. Patient–ventilator asynchrony that causes the patient to attempt to exhale before inspiratory flow stops can also cause an abrupt increase in P_{AW}. In the absence of these two problems, high airway pressure alarms occur almost exclusively when patients are receiving volume control (VC) breaths.

Volume Control Breaths

Figure 6.1 is a plot of P_{AW} and alveolar pressure (P_{ALV}) during a passive VC breath with constant inspiratory flow and PEEP of 5 cmH$_2$O. A brief, end-inspiratory pause is also shown. As discussed in Chapters 1 and 5, at all times during a mechanical breath, P_{AW} is equal to the sum of the pressures needed

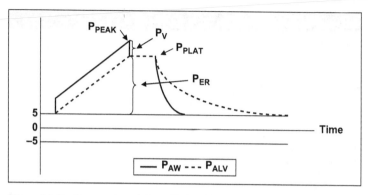

Figure 6.1 Simultaneous plots of airway (P_{AW}) and alveolar (P_{ALV}) pressure versus time during a passive mechanical breath with constant inspiratory flow and 5 cmH$_2$O PEEP. An end-inspiratory pause briefly delays expiration. P_{AW} reaches a peak (P_{PEAK}) at end-inspiration and falls to a plateau pressure (P_{PLAT}) during the end-inspiratory pause. P_{PLAT} is the sum of the elastic recoil pressure generated by the tidal volume (P_{ER}) and total PEEP (PEEP$_T$). The difference between P_{PEAK} and P_{PLAT} is the pressure needed to overcome viscous forces at end-inspiration (P_V).

to overcome viscous forces (P_V), the elastic recoil generated by the delivered volume (P_{ER}), and total end-expiratory pressure (PEEP$_T$). This is expressed mathematically as:

$$P_{AW} = P_V + P_{ER} + PEEP_T \tag{6.1}$$

and as:

$$P_{AW} = (R \times \dot{V}) + (\Delta V/C) + PEEP_T \tag{6.2}$$

If we look only at what determines P_{PEAK} during a VC breath, Equation 6.2 becomes:

$$P_{PEAK} = (R \times \dot{V}_{EI}) + (V_T/C) + PEEP_T \tag{6.3}$$

Here, $\dot{V}_{EI}$ is the flow rate at end-inspiration, and V_T is the delivered tidal volume.

If we have excluded coughing and patient–ventilator asynchrony, the remaining causes of an acute rise in P_{PEAK} are shown by Equation 6.3. If we assume that there hasn't been a recent, unrecognized increase in $\dot{V}_{EI}$, V_T, or extrinsic PEEP, we are left with the causes listed in Box 6.2.

Box 6.2 Causes of High Airway Pressure Alarms During VC Breaths

Increased Pressure Needed to Overcome Viscous Forces (P_V)

• Increased airway resistance
  • Secretions in the large airways or ET tube
  • Kinking of the ET tube
  • Bronchospasm

Increased Pressure Needed to Balance Elastic Recoil (P_{ER})

• Reduced respiratory system compliance
  • Pulmonary edema
• Increased lung volume
  • Right main bronchus intubation
  • Mucous plugging
  • Pneumothorax

Increased Intrinsic PEEP

• Reduced expiratory time
  • Increased spontaneous respiratory rate
• Decreased expiratory flow rate
  • Increased airway resistance, as listed previously

ET = endotracheal; PEEP = positive end-expiratory pressure

That list requires some clarification. First, "increased lung volume" doesn't mean that V_T has increased, but instead that a *portion* of the lungs receives more volume. For example, occlusion of the left main bronchus by mucous or right main bronchus intubation causes the entire tidal volume to enter the right lung. This may or may not reduce lung compliance. If compliance is unchanged, doubling the volume must double the pressure needed to balance the elastic recoil of the right lung. If over-distension leads to a fall in compliance, then P_{ER} will increase even more. Second, the effect of airway secretions depends on the extent of bronchial obstruction. Narrowing of the airway lumen increases resistance and P_V. Complete obstruction, as just mentioned, increases P_{ER}.

So how do you determine which of these problems is responsible for an increase in P_{PEAK}? The first step is to measure P_{AW} during an end-inspiratory pause. As discussed in Chapter 1, when flow stops, viscous forces disappear, and P_{PEAK} rapidly falls to a "plateau" pressure (P_{PLAT}) that equals the total elastic recoil pressure of the respiratory system (P_{ER} + $PEEP_T$). The difference between P_{PEAK} and P_{PLAT} is the pressure needed to overcome viscous forces (P_V) at end-inspiration. You can now determine whether the rise in P_{PEAK} is due to an increase in total elastic recoil or viscous forces.

Figure 6.2 shows the effect of reduced compliance and increased resistance, lung volume, and intrinsic PEEP (PEEP$_I$) on P_{PEAK}, P_{PLAT}, P_V, and P_{ER}. An acute rise in P_{PEAK} that is accompanied by a small $P_{PEAK} - P_{PLAT}$ gradient must be due to a fall in compliance or an increase in lung volume or PEEP$_I$. You can screen for the presence of PEEP$_I$ by examining the flow–time curve on the user interface (Chapters 9 and 10). If each mechanical breath begins before expiratory flow reaches zero, PEEP$_I$ must be present. If P_{PLAT} is much less than P_{PEAK}, there has been an increase in airway resistance.

Appropriate tests must now be performed to diagnose or exclude the causes of increased P_V, P_{ER}, or PEEP$_I$ listed in Box 6.2. As shown in Box 6.3, this evaluation consists of a focused physical examination, a chest radiograph, airway suctioning, and sometimes fiber-optic bronchoscopy. Treatment, of course, depends on the identified cause(s).

Other Types of Mechanical Breaths

Unlike VC breaths, P_{AW} is constant during pressure control (PC), adaptive pressure control (aPC), pressure support (PS), and adaptive pressure support (aPS) breaths, so high airway pressure alarms are almost always due to coughing or patient–ventilator asynchrony. Since P_{AW} increases during aPC and aPS breaths to maintain a clinician-set tidal volume, a high-pressure alarm will occasionally occur if a large increase in P_{AW} is needed to counteract a rise in airway resistance or a fall in compliance or patient inspiratory effort.

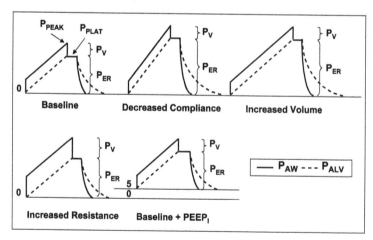

Figure 6.2 The effect of increased volume, resistance, and PEEP$_I$ and reduced compliance on P_{PEAK}, P_{PLAT}, P_V, and P_{ER}.

Box 6.3 Evaluation of High Peak Airway Pressure

Large P_{PEAK}–P_{PLAT} Gradient

- Increased airway resistance
  - Auscultate for rhonchi and wheezing
  - Examine the ET tube for secretions, narrowing, and kinking
  - Assess response of P_{AW} to airway suctioning or bronchoscopy

Small P_{PEAK}–P_{PLAT} Gradient

- Increased lung volume
  - Auscultate for unilateral reduction or loss of breath sounds
  - Examine for asymmetrical chest expansion
  - Examine for tracheal shift, subcutaneous air
  - Obtain CXR to look for right main bronchus intubation, atelectasis, and pneumothorax
- Reduced respiratory system compliance
  - Examine for signs of pulmonary edema and heart failure
  - Obtain CXR to evaluate for pulmonary edema
- Increased intrinsic PEEP
  - Reduced expiratory time
    - Check for recent increase in spontaneous respiratory rate
  - Decreased expiratory flow rate
    - Assess for causes of increased airway resistance, as listed previously

ET = endotracheal; P_{AW} = airway pressure; CXR = chest X-ray; PEEP = positive end-expiratory pressure

Low Airway Pressure

A low airway pressure alarm is triggered whenever P_{AW} falls below a set *low pressure limit*. This is much less common than a high-pressure alarm, but it occurs in two very important situations. The first is when there's a large leak in the ventilator circuit that prevents the set or required P_{AW} from being reached. This most often occurs when the ventilator circuit becomes disconnected from the endotracheal or tracheostomy tube. The second is when the patient's flow requirements exceed the inspiratory flow provided during VC breaths. The greater the difference between the required and the provided flow, the more P_{AW} will fall (see Chapter 5, Figure 5.6).

High Respiratory Rate

This alarm is triggered when the patient's respiratory rate exceeds a *high rate limit* that's typically set 10–15 breaths per minute above the mandatory rate on the CMV and SIMV modes and between 30 and 40 breaths per minute on the spontaneous ventilation mode. The implications of a high respiratory rate alarm differ, depending on the mode of ventilation.

During CMV and SIMV, it means that the patient has a high minute ventilation ($\dot{V}_E$) requirement, that the set mandatory rate is far below the patient's total respiratory rate, and that $\dot{V}_E$ will fall (and $PaCO_2$ will rise) if the patient's respiratory drive decreases (e.g., with sedation). In response, the clinician should determine the cause of the high $\dot{V}_E$ requirement, and, if it cannot be corrected, the mandatory rate should be increased.

During spontaneous ventilation, a marked increase in respiratory rate most often accompanies a drop in tidal volume. This usually results from respiratory muscle fatigue, over-sedation, or both, and indicates that the patient should be returned to the CMV mode.

Low Respiratory Rate

A *low rate limit* is set during spontaneous ventilation. Since there are no mandatory breaths, a low respiratory rate alarm almost always means that the patient is no longer able to maintain adequate $\dot{V}_E$ and must be immediately switched to the CMV mode.

Low Tidal Volume

The *low tidal volume limit* is typically set 150–200 ml less than the set (VC, aPC, aPS) or initially delivered (PC, PS) tidal volume. A low tidal volume alarm is most often precipitated by high airway pressure. Remember that the patient gets little or no ventilation when a high-pressure alarm is active, so naturally, the exhaled tidal volume is very low. This problem is easily recognized when both alarms occur at the same time. Unless it has been caused by a brief coughing spell, the clinician must take immediate steps to diagnose and correct the problem. A low tidal volume alarm will also be triggered by a large leak in the ventilator circuit.

Other causes of a low tidal volume alarm occur only during PC and PS breaths (Box 6.4). Notice that these are the same causes of a high airway pressure alarm during VC breaths (Box 6.2). This is not just a weird coincidence. Remember that VC, aPC, and aPS breaths are volume-set and pressure-variable. If P_V, P_{ER}, or $PEEP_i$ increases, P_{AW} will increase to keep V_T constant. PC and PS breaths are pressure-set and volume-variable. Since P_{AW} cannot increase, a rise in P_V, P_{ER}, or $PEEP_i$ must cause a drop in V_T. Finally, since flow and volume vary with patient inspiratory effort, a low tidal volume alarm may also be triggered by a decrease in respiratory drive or effort, or by respiratory muscle fatigue. This is much more likely to occur during PS breaths, because patient effort is a more important determinant of tidal volume.

When a low tidal volume alarm occurs, the ventilator circuit should be examined for a large air leak. If there is a simultaneous high-pressure alarm, its cause must be identified, as discussed previously. If these problems are ruled

Box 6.4 Causes of Low Tidal Volume Alarms

All Breath Types

• High airway pressure
• Large leak, or ventilator disconnect

Pressure Control and Pressure Support Breaths

• Increased P_V
  • Increased airway resistance
• Increased P_{ER}
  • Increased lung volume
  • Reduced respiratory system compliance
• Increased $PEEP_I$
  • Reduced expiratory time
  • Decreased expiratory flow rate
• Reduced respiratory drive or effort

P_V = pressure required to overcome viscous forces; P_{ER} = pressure required to overcome the increase in elastic recoil produced by the tidal volume; $PEEP_I$ = intrinsic PEEP

out, patients receiving PC or PS breaths should be evaluated with a focused physical examination, chest radiograph, and, if necessary, fiber-optic bronchoscopy. Not surprisingly, the evaluation for a low tidal volume alarm and a high airway pressure alarm are the same (Box 6.3).

Section 3

Patient Management

In the final section of this book, you'll learn how to use your knowledge of pulmonary and cardiovascular physiology and the "nuts and bolts" of mechanical ventilators to expertly manage critically ill, mechanically ventilated patients. This section will cover the indications for intubation and mechanical ventilation, how to write ventilator orders, how to assess your patient while they're on the ventilator, and how to identify and manage dynamic hyperinflation and patient–ventilator asynchrony. It will also review ventilator management in patients with several particularly challenging diseases; specifically, acute respiratory distress syndrome (ARDS), severe obstructive lung disease, and right ventricular failure. Finally, you will get lots of information about discontinuing or "weaning" mechanical ventilation and how and when to use "noninvasive" ventilation.

Chapter 7

Respiratory Failure and the Indications for Mechanical Ventilation

Chapters 1 and 2 explained how the respiratory system maintains a normal arterial partial pressure of oxygen (PaO_2) and carbon dioxide ($PaCO_2$). *Respiratory failure* occurs when a disease process significantly interferes with this vital function and causes arterial hypoxemia, hypercapnia, or both. Typically, respiratory failure is divided into three categories, based on the underlying pathophysiology:

- Ventilation failure
- Oxygenation failure
- Oxygenation-ventilation failure

With severe disturbances in gas exchange, mechanical ventilation is often needed to assist the respiratory system and restore the $PaCO_2$, PaO_2, or both, to normal.

Respiratory Failure

Ventilation Failure

As defined in this chapter, *ventilation failure* is caused by a *primary decrease in minute ventilation* ($\dot{V}_E$) that prevents the respiratory system from maintaining a normal $PaCO_2$. Recall this equation from Chapter 2:

$$PaCO_2 \propto \dot{V}_PCO_2/\dot{V}_E - \dot{V}_D \tag{7.1}$$

It tells us that, for a given level of CO_2 production ($\dot{V}_PCO_2$) and dead space ventilation ($\dot{V}_D$), $PaCO_2$ varies inversely with $\dot{V}_E$. As $\dot{V}_E$ falls, $PaCO_2$ rises.

As shown in Table 7.1, $\dot{V}_E$ can be reduced by any disease that decreases central respiratory drive, interferes with the transmission of neural signals from the brain to the respiratory muscles, or reduces respiratory muscle strength. Inadequate $\dot{V}_E$ can also be caused by disorders such as morbid obesity and severe kyphoscoliosis, which reduce chest wall compliance and increase the pressure that must be generated by the respiratory muscles.

Table 7.1 Causes of Ventilation Failure

Category	Causes	Examples
Reduced respiratory drive	Drugs and toxins	Narcotics, sedatives
	Metabolic encephalopathy	Liver failure, renal failure
	Encephalitis/Meningitis	
	Cerebral or brainstem infarction	
	Intracranial hemorrhage	
Impaired transmission to the respiratory muscles	Spinal cord disease	Trauma, myelitis, ALS
	Peripheral neuropathy	Phrenic nerve injury, Guillain-Barre syndrome
	Disease of the neuromuscular junction	Myasthenia gravis, Eaton-Lambert syndrome
Respiratory muscle weakness	Myopathy	Endocrine, metabolic, drug-induced
	Myositis	Polymyositis, other connective tissue diseases
Chest wall disease	Reduced chest wall compliance	Morbid obesity, severe kyphoscoliosis, large pleural effusions, massive ascites

ALS = amyotrophic lateral sclerosis

Since the diseases that precipitate ventilation failure do not affect the lungs themselves, they do not increase the normal degree of mismatching between ventilation ($\dot{V}$) and perfusion ($\dot{Q}$) or affect the normal distribution of $\dot{V}/\dot{Q}$ ratios.[1] This means that the mean alveolar PO_2 ($P\bar{A}O_2$) calculated from the alveolar gas equation (Chapter 2, Equation 2.4) and the measured PaO_2 fall together with the rise in $PaCO_2$, and the difference between them (the A–a gradient) does not change (see Table 7.3).

Oxygenation Failure

Oxygenation failure occurs when *intrinsic lung disease* causes a drop in the PaO_2 and arterial hemoglobin saturation (SaO_2). As discussed in Chapter 2, this results from the generation of abnormal $\dot{V}/\dot{Q}$ ratios (including intra-pulmonary shunting), the impairment of gas diffusion, or both. As shown in Table 7.2, oxygenation failure can be caused by any lung disease, regardless of whether it primarily affects the airways, the lung parenchyma, or the pulmonary circulation. Since lung disease does not alter any of the components of the alveolar gas equation, the calculated $P\bar{A}O_2$ is unchanged, and the A–a gradient increases (see Table 7.3). Recall that an abnormal degree of $\dot{V}/\dot{Q}$ mismatching and diffusion impairment can also cause hypercapnia. In patients with oxygenation failure, an appropriate increase in $\dot{V}_E$ mediated by central chemoreceptors maintains a normal $PaCO_2$.

---

1 This will only be true if impaired ventilation does not lead to lung atelectasis.

Table 7.2 Causes of Oxygenation Failure

Category	Examples
Obstructive lung diseases	Emphysema
	Chronic bronchitis
	Asthma
	Bronchiectasis
Restrictive lung diseases	Idiopathic pulmonary fibrosis
	Sarcoidosis
	Pneumoconioses
Airspace filling diseases	ARDS
	Cardiogenic edema
	Pneumonia
Pulmonary vascular diseases	Pulmonary arterial hypertension
	Pulmonary embolism

ARDS = acute respiratory distress syndrome

Oxygenation-Ventilation Failure

It will probably come as no surprise that this type of respiratory failure combines the features of both oxygenation and ventilation failure. Its pathophysiology is largely the same as pure oxygenation failure. The difference is that the underlying lung disease causes such a profound abnormality in lung compliance or resistance that the respiratory system either cannot maintain a normal $\dot{V}_E$ or it cannot increase $\dot{V}_E$ to compensate for hypercapnia caused by $\dot{V}/\dot{Q}$ mismatching or diffusion impairment. As shown in Table 7.3, patients with oxygenation-ventilation failure have a reduced PaO_2, an elevated $PaCO_2$, and an increased A–a gradient. In theory, any of the diseases listed in Table 7.2 can lead to oxygenation-ventilation failure, but the most common causes are the acute respiratory distress syndrome (ARDS), cardiogenic pulmonary edema, chronic obstructive pulmonary disease (COPD), and severe acute asthma.

Acute, Chronic, and Acute-on-Chronic Hypercapnia

Hypercapnia in patients with either ventilation failure or oxygenation-ventilation failure can occur quickly over a period of minutes to hours, or develop gradually over weeks, months, or years. Chronic hypercapnia leads

Table 7.3 Diagnostic Features of Respiratory Failure

	PaO_2	$PaCO_2$	A–a Gradient
Ventilation failure	↓	↑	NL
Oxygenation failure	↓	NL or ↓	↑
Oxygenation-ventilation failure	↓	↑	↑

NL = normal

to renal compensation, which increases the serum bicarbonate concentration and returns the arterial pH toward normal. That's why the terms "acute" and "chronic" also imply differences in clinical manifestations and in the urgency of therapy. Patients with chronic, compensated hypercapnia may also develop an acute decompensation that worsens respiratory acidosis. This is referred to as "acute-on-chronic" hypercapnia.

Indications for Mechanical Ventilation

There are four indications for intubation and mechanical ventilation:

- Acute or acute-on-chronic hypercapnia
- Oxygenation failure with refractory hypoxemia
- Inability to protect the lower airway
- Upper airway obstruction

Acute or Acute-on-Chronic Hypercapnia

Hypercapnia itself is rarely dangerous. It's the accompanying acidemia (low arterial pH) that may cause major morbidity or even death. So it's the patient with acute or acute-on-chronic ventilation or oxygenation-ventilation failure that often needs mechanical ventilation, not the patient with chronic, compensated respiratory acidosis from, say, long-standing COPD or morbid obesity.

As a rule of thumb, patients with hypercapnia-induced acidemia should be intubated when their arterial pH falls below about 7.20. Recognize, though, that this is a very general guideline, and that clinical judgment must always prevail. For example, earlier intubation is usually advisable in patients whose hypercapnia and arterial pH are steadily worsening despite aggressive therapy.

In many cases, in fact, patients with respiratory distress are intubated *before* any change in $PaCO_2$ or pH has occurred. That's because early intubation for *impending* hypercapnia is much safer than waiting until the onset of respiratory muscle fatigue, which can precipitate acute, severe, and life-threatening acidemia. On the other hand, a patient with a pH < 7.20 may not require intubation if the cause can be rapidly corrected (e.g., narcotic-induced ventilation failure). Also keep in mind that the decision to intubate a patient is often made in the absence of blood gas measurements. For instance, an unresponsive patient who is taking very slow and shallow breaths should be immediately intubated and ventilated without waiting to confirm the presence of severe hypercapnia and acidemia.

Refractory Hypoxemia

In most patients, oxygenation failure can be adequately treated simply by providing oxygen through a nasal cannula or face mask. Intubation and mechanical ventilation are needed only when the PaO_2 and SaO_2 remain *critically low* despite high-flow supplemental oxygen. This is referred to as "refractory hypoxemia" and typically occurs in patients with ARDS, cardiogenic edema, and other diseases that cause extensive alveolar filling. Here, my use of the term "critically low" is intentionally vague. Although a PaO_2 > 60 mmHg and an SaO_2 > 90% are reasonable goals, there's no generally accepted PaO_2 or SaO_2 that mandates intubation, and decisions must be made on a case-by-case basis.

So why is mechanical ventilation beneficial to patients with refractory hypoxemia? After all, their $PaCO_2$ is usually normal or low, so they don't need assistance with ventilation. The main advantage is that endotracheal intubation allows us to go from an *open* to a *closed* system of oxygen delivery. Patients receiving supplemental oxygen via a face mask always inhale a variable volume of room air. This causes the fractional concentration of *inspired* oxygen (F_iO_2) to be less than the concentration of O_2 flowing to the patient (FO_2). Following intubation, though, the cuff of the endotracheal tube prevents room air from entering. This means that an F_iO_2 of 1.0, or any other concentration, can be reliably delivered, and this is usually accompanied by a significant improvement in PaO_2 and SaO_2.

The other benefit of mechanical ventilation is that it allows the use of positive end-expiratory pressure. As discussed in several previous chapters, by maintaining positive (supra-atmospheric) pressure in the airways and alveoli throughout expiration, PEEP prevents alveoli that were opened or "recruited" during mechanical inflation from collapsing during expiration. This reduces the volume of blood passing through unventilated alveoli (intra-pulmonary shunt) and improves oxygenation.

Inability to Protect the Lower Airway

Normally, several very effective mechanisms prevent saliva, food, and liquids from entering the trachea. During spontaneous breathing, the true and false vocal folds are abducted (separated), the entrance to the trachea (glottis) is open, and air passes freely in and out of the tracheobronchial tree. If saliva or another substance enters the larynx, reflexes mediated via the vagus nerve immediately adduct (bring together) the vocal folds and close the glottis. If aspiration does occur, irritant receptors in the larynx and trachea trigger a powerful cough response that forces the material back up through the glottis. When we swallow, there are two barriers to aspiration. First, the vocal folds adduct and close the glottis. (That's why we can't breathe and swallow at the same time). Second, the larynx is pulled upward toward the base of the tongue, which pushes the epiglottis downward like a protective cover over the laryngeal inlet.

Endotracheal intubation is commonly performed when a patient is believed to have lost these vital protective reflexes. But there are two big problems. Problem #1: How do you know when patients are unable to "protect their airway"? Usually, this is based on the assumption that the patient's mental status predicts the effectiveness of their protective reflexes. Although this makes sense and a general correlation is supported by some observational studies, the actual relationship between the level of consciousness and the presence of airway protective reflexes is simply unknown. In other words, we don't know what proportion of comatose, obtunded, or lethargic patients cannot protect themselves from aspiration. Compounding this problem is the fact that bedside assessments are unreliable. In particular, most studies have shown a poor correlation between the presence or absence of a gag reflex and protective laryngeal reflexes.

Why is this so important? Isn't it just better to intubate a patient with altered mental status and make sure that their airway is protected? Well, this brings us to Problem #2. I want you to consider what happens to normal protective reflexes when a patient is intubated. The patient is now unable to close the glottis, elevate the larynx, or cough. In other words, all protective reflexes have been eliminated. In fact, saliva can (and does) freely flow into the trachea between the endotracheal tube and the vocal folds. But doesn't the cuff of the endotracheal tube still protect the lower airway? It protects against acute, large-volume (massive) aspiration, but saliva and other substances eventually pass around the cuff and enter the tracheobronchial tree. In fact, this is the pathogenesis of ventilator-associated pneumonia.

So, as you can see, intubating a patient to "protect" their lower airway is sometimes the wrong thing to do, because it prevents intact laryngeal reflexes from functioning. We just don't know when it's the wrong thing to do. Based on everything I've told you, I intubate patients for airway protection under two circumstances. The first is when a condition that is not quickly reversible causes the patient to be completely unresponsive or responsive only to painful stimuli. The second is when a patient who is having or is likely to have large-volume emesis (e.g., gastric outlet or small bowel obstruction, upper GI bleeding) has even a modest decline in his or her level of consciousness.

Upper Airway Obstruction

This is the most obvious but least common indication for intubation and mechanical ventilation. When narrowing of the pharynx or larynx prevents adequate ventilation, it must be bypassed with an artificial airway. This can usually be accomplished with an endotracheal tube, but tracheostomy may be needed when there is marked anatomical distortion or complete airway obstruction.

Chapter 8

How to Write Ventilator Orders

Now that you've learned all about ventilator terminology, modes and breath types, and the indications for mechanical ventilation, you're ready to write ventilator orders. As you'll see, this is really pretty easy, but it's important that you take an orderly, step-by-step approach.

This chapter is divided into three sections:

- Initial ventilator orders—How to choose appropriate settings immediately after intubation
- Adjusting ventilator settings—How to make changes throughout the course of your patient's illness
- Weaning from mechanical ventilation—How to write orders for "spontaneous breathing trials"

Initial Ventilator Orders

Step 1: Choose a Mode of Mechanical Ventilation

As discussed in Chapter 5, the CMV mode is ideal for critically ill patients with respiratory failure because it guarantees a clinician-set number of mechanical breaths, allows the patient to control the total respiratory rate, and requires very little patient inspiratory effort and work of breathing.

My recommendation:

- Always use CMV as the initial mode of mechanical ventilation.

Step 2: Choose the Type of Mechanical Breath

Here you get to choose between five breath types (described in Chapter 5): volume control (VC), pressure control (PC), adaptive pressure control (aPC), pressure support (PS), and adaptive pressure support (aPS). I prefer to initially use VC or aPC breaths in all patients because they provide a clinician-set tidal volume. The combination of VC or aPC breaths with the CMV mode guarantees a minimum, safe minute ventilation.

My recommendation:

- Use VC or aPC breaths with the CMV mode.

Step 3: Select Settings Based on the Type of Mechanical Breath

Remember that each breath type requires you to set specific parameters. So, your next set of orders depends on whether you've picked VC or aPC breaths in Step 2. If you chose VC breaths, you must specify the delivered tidal volume (V_T) and, depending on the ventilator, set either the peak inspiratory flow and the flow profile or the inspiratory time (T_I). If you selected aPC breaths, you have to set the V_T and T_I.

My recommendations:

- VC breaths
  - Tidal volume:
    ~ 8 ml/kg ideal body weight (IBW)
    ≤ 6 ml/kg IBW in patients with the acute respiratory distress syndrome
  - Peak inspiratory flow: 60–80 L/min
  - Flow profile: Descending ramp
  - Inspiratory time: 0.6–0.8 second
- aPC breaths
  - Tidal volume: Same as for VC breaths
  - Inspiratory time: Same as for VC breaths

Step 4: Specify Other Basic Settings

Fractional Inspired Oxygen Concentration (F_IO_2)
Hypoxemia is bad! Always start with a high F_IO_2 and decrease it later, if possible. Never start low and work your way up.

My recommendations:

- Patients with a high oxygen requirement prior to intubation should initially receive an F_IO_2 of 1.0.
- In patients with acute or acute-on-chronic hypercapnia and modest oxygen requirements, an initial F_IO_2 of 0.5 is usually okay.

Mandatory Respiratory Rate (RR)
This is the number of guaranteed breaths each minute, and it must be specified in the CMV and SIMV modes.

My recommendations:

- As a general rule, the mandatory rate should initially be set between 10 and 14 breaths per minute.
- Patients with chronic hypercapnia may only need 6–10 breaths per minute.

Positive End-Expiratory Pressure (PEEP)
PEEP is used to help open or "recruit" atelectatic alveoli and improve PaO_2 in patients with extensive alveolar filling. In many hospitals, a small amount of PEEP (e.g., 5 cmH$_2$O) is routinely used in all mechanically ventilated patients to prevent atelectasis.

My recommendations:

- Patients with severe air flow obstruction are likely to have dynamic hyperinflation and intrinsic PEEP. Set PEEP at zero for these patients.
- In all other patients, start at a PEEP of 5.0 cmH$_2$O.

Trigger Type

Very sensitive techniques have shown that, when compared with pressure-triggering, flow-triggering decreases the time between the onset of patient inspiratory effort and gas entry into the lungs and reduces patient work of breathing. The magnitude of this difference, though, does not appear to be clinically relevant, and these two triggering methods should be considered interchangeable. Refer to Chapter 4 for a review of pressure and flow-triggering.

My recommendation:

- Select either pressure or flow triggering.

Trigger Sensitivity

The effort required to trigger the ventilator increases as pressure sensitivity becomes more negative and flow sensitivity becomes more positive. Ideally, sensitivity is set to allow easy triggering with low risk of auto-triggering (see Chapter 11).

My recommendations:

- Set pressure sensitivity at –1 or –2 cmH$_2$O.
- Set flow sensitivity at 1 or 2 L/min.

Summary

Table 8.1 provides an example of initial ventilator orders.

Table 8.1 Initial Ventilator Orders

Ventilator mode:	CMV
Breath type:	VC or aPC
Tidal volume:	500 ml
Inspiratory time:*	0.7 seconds
Peak flow:*	60 L/min
Flow profile:*	Descending ramp
F$_I$O$_2$:	1.0 or 0.5
Mandatory rate:	12 breaths/minute
PEEP:	5 cmH$_2$O
Trigger type:	Pressure
Sensitivity:	–2 cmH$_2$O

* Set either inspiratory time or peak flow and profile depending on the ventilator.

CMV = continuous mandatory ventilation; VC = volume control; aPC = adaptive pressure control

Adjusting Ventilator Settings

After you write your initial orders, you'll need to make adjustments during the time your patient is on the ventilator. Most will be in response to one or more of the following conditions: high or low PaO_2 and SpO_2, respiratory acidosis, or respiratory alkalosis.

High PaO_2 and SpO_2

If you follow my recommendation and start with a high F_iO_2, you'll often need to reduce it after your first arterial blood gas (ABG) measurements. You will also be able to decrease the F_iO_2 as your patient's underlying lung disease improves. You should reduce the F_iO_2 as much as possible, while keeping the PaO_2 between about 70 and 80 mmHg. Unfortunately, there's no reliable way to predict what effect a decrease in the F_iO_2 will have.

That's because the relationship between the F_iO_2 and PaO_2 depends on the type and severity of the underlying gas exchange abnormality. As shown in Figure 8.1A, $\dot{V}/\dot{Q}$ mismatching causes a curvilinear relationship that varies with the severity and extent of disease. Notice that even when $\dot{V}/\dot{Q}$ imbalance is severe, PaO_2 increases dramatically at high F_iO_2. That's because, as long as some ventilation is present, even very low $\dot{V}/\dot{Q}$ alveoli will eventually fill with O_2, and the blood leaving them will have a high PO_2 and hemoglobin saturation.

When intrapulmonary shunting is present, some alveoli receive no ventilation. Increasing the F_iO_2 has no effect on the shunted blood and, above a certain level, cannot further increase the saturation of blood passing through ventilated alveoli. This produces a linear relationship between PaO_2 and F_iO_2 (Figure 8.1B) that flattens as the *shunt fraction* (the percentage of the cardiac output flowing through unventilated alveoli) increases.

Since lung disease often produces both $\dot{V}/\dot{Q}$ mismatching and shunt, there's no way to predict the PaO_2–F_iO_2 relationship in a particular patient. So, here's what you do. First, make sure that the hemoglobin saturation measured by pulse oximetry (SpO_2) is accurate by comparing it with the saturation measured from an ABG (SaO_2). If it is, simply reduce the F_iO_2 in small increments until the SpO_2 is consistently around 93%. I like to shoot for 93% because, even under the best of circumstances, the SpO_2 may be off by 2%. Further decreases in the F_iO_2 should be based on PaO_2 and SaO_2 measurements.

Low PaO_2 and SpO_2

If your patient has extensive airspace filling, it's likely that, at some time during the course of their illness, the PaO_2 and SpO_2 will be low even when they're receiving high F_iO_2. At that point, the first step is to gradually increase the level of PEEP. By increasing mean alveolar pressure, PEEP opens

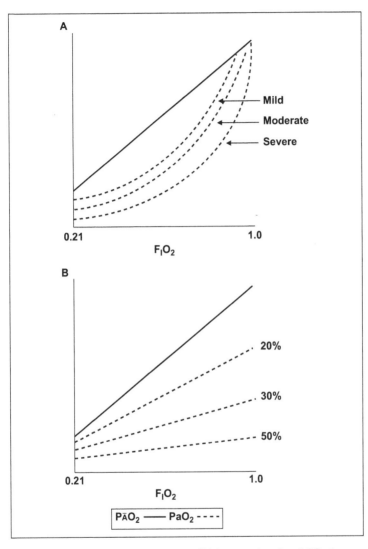

Figure 8.1 The calculated mean alveolar PO_2 ($P\bar{A}O_2$) increases linearly with F_IO_2. As the severity of $\dot{V}/\dot{Q}$ mismatching increases (A), the relationship between the fractional concentration of inspired oxygen (F_IO_2) and the arterial partial pressure of oxygen (PaO_2) becomes increasingly curvilinear. In the presence of a right-to-left shunt (B), there is a linear relationship between F_IO_2 and PaO_2. As shunt fraction (expressed as percent of cardiac output) increases, there is a smaller and smaller rise in PaO_2 with F_IO_2.

or "recruits" atelectatic alveoli and reduces intra-pulmonary shunting. In general, PaO_2 increases with increments in PEEP; but be careful. As discussed in Chapter 3, PEEP reduces venous return and increases RV afterload, which can significantly decrease LV preload, cardiac output, and tissue O_2 delivery. I suggest that you increase PEEP in increments of 3–5 cmH$_2$O while monitoring stroke volume or cardiac output, or at least watching closely for signs of impaired tissue perfusion. PEEP levels over 20 cmH$_2$O are rarely used. PEEP and other ways of increasing PaO_2, including prone positioning, neuromuscular blockade, and inhaled vasodilators, are discussed in detail in Chapter 12.

Respiratory Acidosis

In Chapter 2, you learned that hypercapnia and respiratory acidosis occur when alveolar ventilation is insufficient to excrete the CO_2 produced by the body, and that this can result from low minute ventilation ($\dot{V}_E$), high dead space ventilation ($\dot{V}_D$), or high CO_2 production ($\dot{V}_PCO_2$).

$$PaCO_2 \propto \dot{V}_PCO_2 / (\dot{V}_E - \dot{V}_D) \qquad (8.1)$$

When caring for critically ill patients, there's typically little you can do to significantly reduce $\dot{V}_PCO_2$ or $\dot{V}_D$, so, regardless of the underlying cause, your response to respiratory acidosis must be to increase $\dot{V}_E$. You could do this using a trial-and-error approach and gradually increase $\dot{V}_E$ while following serial ABGs, but there's a better way. If we make the reasonable assumption that $\dot{V}_PCO_2$ and $\dot{V}_D$ remain constant over a short period of time, then $PaCO_2$ is inversely related to $\dot{V}_E$, and Equation 8.1 becomes:

$$PaCO_2 \propto 1/\dot{V}_E \qquad (8.2)$$

We can then set up a proportion between the current $PaCO_2$ ($PaCO_2$-1) and $\dot{V}_E$($\dot{V}_E$-1), and the $\dot{V}_E$ needed ($\dot{V}_E$-2) to give the $PaCO_2$ that we want ($PaCO_2$-2).

$$PaCO_2\text{-}1 \times \dot{V}_E\text{-}1 = PaCO_2\text{-}2 \times \dot{V}_E\text{-}2 \qquad (8.3)$$

and

$$PaCO_2\text{-}1 / \dot{V}_E\text{-}2 = PaCO_2\text{-}2 / \dot{V}_E\text{-}1 \qquad (8.4)$$

If tidal volume isn't changed[1], we can substitute respiratory rate (RR) for $\dot{V}_E$ and rewrite this equation as:

$$PaCO_2\text{-}1/RR\text{-}2 = PaCO_2\text{-}2/RR\text{-}1 \qquad (8.5)$$

Solving for RR-2 gives us

$$RR\text{-}2 = \left(PaCO_2\text{-}1 / PaCO_2\text{-}2\right) \times RR\text{-}1 \qquad (8.6)$$

So, let's say that a patient is being ventilated at a rate of 10 breaths per minute and has a $PaCO_2$ of 65 mmHg. The rate needed to reduce the $PaCO_2$ to 40 mmHg is (65/40) x 10, or about 16 breaths per minute. When doing these calculations, it's important to recognize that it takes a while to see the full effect of a change in ventilation. That's because the body contains an enormous store of CO_2 (about 120 L) that exists in a variety of different forms. So wait for at least 20 minutes before checking to see if the change in respiratory rate was effective.

Respiratory Alkalosis

Hypocapnia and respiratory alkalosis occur when minute ventilation exceeds that needed to maintain a normal $PaCO_2$. This may be due to patient agitation or discomfort, and in these cases, the problem often resolves with appropriate sedation or analgesia. Much more often though, respiratory alkalosis occurs simply because the mandatory rate has been set too high. You can easily distinguish between these two possibilities by comparing the set and total respiratory rates displayed on the user interface of the ventilator. If they're the same, the patient's respiratory alkalosis is iatrogenic, and you need to reduce the set rate. You can use the method we just discussed to calculate the rate needed to return the $PaCO_2$ and pH to normal, or you can simply decrease the set rate until the patient begins to trigger spontaneous breaths.

Weaning from Mechanical Ventilation

Once the underlying cause of respiratory failure has resolved or significantly improved, you need to determine whether or not your patient is ready for

---

1 Recall from Chapter 2 that any change in V_T changes the $\dot{V}_E$ needed to maintain a given $PaCO_2$ because it alters the ratio of dead space to tidal volume (V_D/V_T). That's why we always change RR rather than V_T.

Table 8.2 Orders for a Spontaneous Breathing Trial

Ventilator mode	Spontaneous ventilation
Breath type:	PS
Pressure support level:	5 cmH$_2$O
PEEP:	0 or 5 cmH$_2$O
F$_i$O$_2$:	Same as on CMV
Trigger type:	Pressure
Sensitivity:	−2 cmH$_2$O

PS = pressure support

extubation. This is most often done by evaluating a number of parameters, including tidal volume, respiratory rate, and vital capacity during so-called spontaneous breathing trials. These trials can be truly spontaneous; that is, the patient is disconnected from the ventilator, or they can be performed using low-level pressure support breaths. I prefer the latter approach because it maintains functioning ventilator alarms, compensates for the extra work needed to breathe through the endotracheal tube, and eliminates the need to disconnect and reconnect the patient.

Table 8.2 shows the orders needed to perform an on-ventilator spontaneous breathing trial. Chapter 15 provides an in-depth discussion about how to discontinue mechanical ventilation.

Chapter 9

Physiological Assessment of the Mechanically Ventilated Patient

In Chapters 1 and 2, I reviewed the essential aspects of pulmonary physiology and discussed how the respiratory system uses the interrelated processes of ventilation and gas exchange to maintain a normal partial pressure of oxygen (PaO_2) and carbon dioxide ($PaCO_2$) in the arterial blood. Recall that the essential components of normal ventilation and gas exchange are:

- Delivery of oxygen
- Excretion of carbon dioxide
- Matching of ventilation and perfusion
- Gas diffusion

As I discussed in Chapter 7, disease-induced abnormalities of one or more of these components cause respiratory failure, which can be divided into oxygenation, ventilation, and oxygenation-ventilation failure, based on the PaO_2 and $PaCO_2$ and the difference between the calculated mean alveolar and measured arterial PO_2 (the A–a gradient). This chapter reviews the tests that can be used to determine the type and severity of respiratory failure and the extent to which one or more of the components of normal ventilation and gas exchange have been compromised by disease.

PaO_2 and SaO_2

The simplest way to determine how much lung disease has interfered with normal gas exchange is to measure the PaO_2 and arterial hemoglobin saturation (SaO_2). The arterial hemoglobin saturation is the ratio of O_2-carrying hemoglobin (oxyhemoglobin; O_2Hb) to total hemoglobin (THb) and is usually expressed as a percentage.

$$SaO_2 = (O_2Hb/THb) \times 100 \qquad (9.1)$$

Total hemoglobin consists of oxyhemoglobin, deoxygenated hemoglobin (HHb), and abnormal hemoglobins, including methemoglobin (MetHb) and carboxyhemoglobin (COHb), which are normally present in very small quantities.

Arterial hemoglobin saturation is measured from an arterial blood sample using a technique called *co-oximetry*, which takes advantage of the fact that each form of hemoglobin has its own light-absorption profile or spectrum (Figure 9.1). Co-oximetry generates a minimum of four different wavelengths of light, which allows it to distinguish between the various forms of hemoglobin based on their absorbance patterns. By measuring the fraction of each wavelength that is absorbed by and transmitted through a hemolyzed blood sample, the concentration of each form of hemoglobin can be accurately measured, and SaO_2 can be calculated as:

$$SaO_2 = O_2Hb/(O_2Hb + HHb + MetHb + COHb) \times 100 \qquad (9.2)$$

The relationship between PaO_2 and SaO_2 is shown by the *oxygen–hemoglobin dissociation curve* (Figure 9.2). Because of its well-known sigmoidal shape, SaO_2 changes relatively little once the PaO_2 exceeds 60–70 mmHg, but below this level, even small changes in the PaO_2 have large effects on the SaO_2. As shown in Figure 9.2, the curve shifts to the right as body temperature increases and blood pH falls, and SaO_2 decreases at a given PaO_2. Hypothermia and alkalemia cause the curve to shift in the opposite direction.

Be careful! Co-oximetry is not used by all blood gas laboratories. Sometimes SaO_2 is calculated from the measured PaO_2 by using the predicted

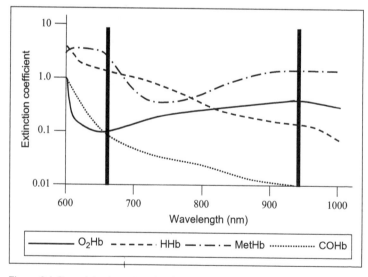

Figure 9.1 Plots of the absorption of oxyhemoglobin (O_2HB), deoxygenated hemoglobin (HHB), methemoglobin (MetHb), and carboxyhemoglobin (COHb). The wavelengths used by pulse oximetry (660 and 940 nm) are shown by the black bars.

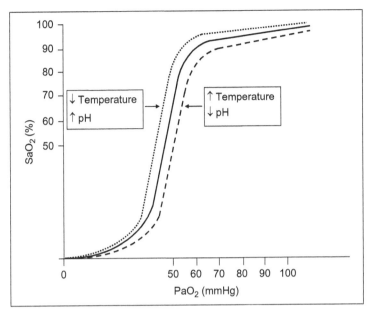

Figure 9.2 The relationship between the arterial partial pressure of oxygen (PaO₂) and the hemoglobin saturation (SaO₂). The curve shifts with changes in body temperature and blood pH.

oxygen–hemoglobin dissociation curve. This technique is subject to a number of errors, the most important being the assumption that there are negligible amounts of MetHb and COHb.

Pulse Oximetry

Like co-oximetry, pulse oximetry calculates arterial hemoglobin saturation by measuring the amount of light absorbed and transmitted by the arterial blood. There are two important technical differences, though. First, pulse oximeters use only two wavelengths of light, which correspond to the maximum absorption of oxyhemoglobin (940 nM) and deoxygenated hemoglobin (660 nM) (Figure 9.1). Second, light is transmitted through tissue (usually a fingertip) rather than a hemolyzed blood sample. This requires software to determine the amount of each wavelength absorbed by the pulsatile arterial blood while factoring out absorption by tissue and venous blood. The hemoglobin saturation, which is referred to as the SpO₂, is determined by comparing the absorption ratio of these two wavelengths with a stored set of reference values.

The advantage of pulse oximetry, of course, is that it can noninvasively and continuously measure and display the arterial hemoglobin saturation. When everything goes right, the SpO_2 is usually within ±2% of the SaO_2 measured by co-oximetry. Unfortunately, several patient-related factors may lead to significant errors.

First, pulse oximetry is often inaccurate in patients with hypotension or poor peripheral perfusion because of its inability to detect and isolate absorption by pulsatile blood. Although most oximeters generate a plethysmographic pulse tracing, a normal-appearing waveform, while helpful, does not guarantee an accurate SpO_2 under these conditions. Since pulse oximeters only measure oxyhemoglobin and deoxygenated hemoglobin, a second problem is that significant errors occur when abnormal amounts of MetHb or COHb are present. Methemoglobin absorbs light at both 940 nm and 660 nm (Figure 9.1). The net result is that SpO_2 falls with increasing MetHb concentration but then plateaus at about 85–88%. This causes pulse oximetry to overestimate the true hemoglobin saturation at high MetHb concentrations. Since carboxyhemoglobin and oxyhemoglobin have very similar absorption at 660 nm, SpO_2 usually remains normal even at high COHb concentrations. Finally, it's not uncommon to see significant and totally unexplained differences between SpO_2 and SaO_2. Because of these problems, I recommend that you routinely confirm the accuracy of SpO_2 readings by measuring SaO_2 every day or two. More frequent measurements are appropriate for patients with hypotension, poor perfusion, abnormal plethysmographic tracings, or markedly impaired oxygenation.

The Alveolar to Arterial PO$_2$ Gradient

Also referred to as the A–a gradient, this is the difference between the mean alveolar PO_2 ($P\overline{A}O_2$) and the measured PaO_2. As discussed in Chapter 2, $P\overline{A}O_2$ is calculated using the alveolar gas equation:

$$P\overline{A}O_2 = \left(P_B - P_{H2O}\right) \times F_IO_2 - \left(P\overline{A}CO_2/R\right) \tag{9.3}$$

In this equation, P_B is barometric pressure, P_{H2O} is the partial pressure of water in the lungs (47 mmHg), F_IO_2 is the fractional concentration of O_2 entering the lungs, $P\overline{A}CO_2$ is the mean alveolar PCO_2 (assumed to equal the $PaCO_2$), and R is the respiratory quotient (assumed to be 0.8). Since the F_IO_2 must be known, the A–a gradient can be calculated only if the patient is breathing room air ($F_IO_2 = 0.21$) or receiving a known F_IO_2 through a closed system (i.e., an endotracheal tube).

Remember that if the lungs were "perfect," every alveolus would have the same ventilation–perfusion ($\dot{V}/\dot{Q}$) ratio, $P\overline{A}O_2$ and PaO_2 would be equal, and the A–a gradient would be zero. In the presence of ventilation–perfusion mismatching, low $\dot{V}/\dot{Q}$ alveoli and shunt cause the PaO_2 to fall without altering the calculated $P\bar{A}O_2$, and the A–a gradient rises. Since even normal lungs have mismatching of ventilation and perfusion as well as a small amount of intra-pulmonary shunting, the normal A–a gradient is about 6–10 mmHg. In the presence of lung disease, the A–a gradient increases with the number of low $\dot{V}/\dot{Q}$ and unventilated alveoli.

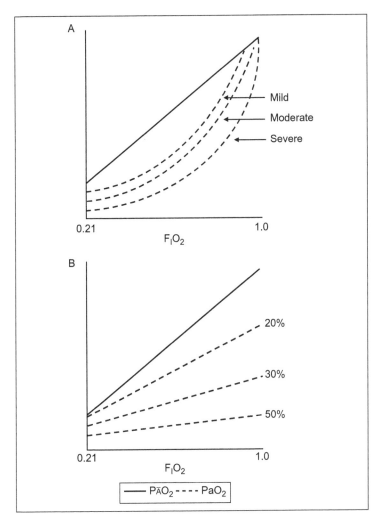

Figure 9.3 Plots of mean alveolar ($P\bar{A}O_2$) and arterial (PaO_2) oxygen partial pressure versus the fractional inspired O_2 concentration (F_iO_2) with (A) varying degrees of $\dot{V}/\dot{Q}$ inequality (mild, moderate, and severe) and (B) percent shunt.

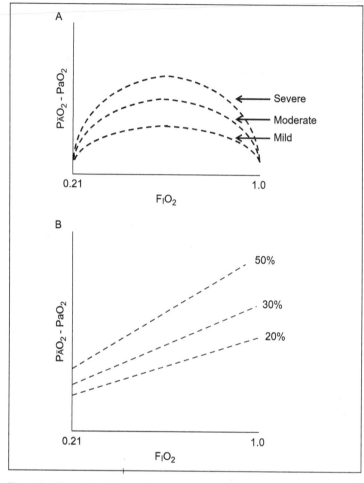

Figure 9.4 Plots of the difference between mean alveolar ($P\overline{A}O_2$) and arterial (PaO_2) oxygen partial pressure versus fractional inspired oxygen concentration (F_IO_2) with varying degrees of (A) $\dot{V}/\dot{Q}$ inequality (mild, moderate, and severe) and (B) percent shunt. With $\dot{V}/\dot{Q}$ inequality alone, the A–a gradient peaks in the mid-F_IO_2 range. When shunt is present, the A–a gradient progressively increases with F_IO_2.

Although there's a general correlation between the A–a gradient and the extent of lung disease, its usefulness as a measure of disease severity is limited by its dependence on F_IO_2 and the underlying gas exchange abnormality. Recall from Chapter 8 that $\dot{V}/\dot{Q}$ mismatching causes a curvilinear relationship between F_IO_2 and PaO_2 that varies with the severity and extent of disease

(Figure 9.3A). Since $P\overline{A}O_2$ increases linearly with F_IO_2 (Equation 9.3), you can see that the A–a gradient must first rise and then fall as the F_IO_2 is increased from 0.21 to 1.0 (Figure 9.4A). On the other hand, when intrapulmonary shunting predominates (Figure 9.3B), the PaO_2–F_IO_2 relationship is linear, and its slope decreases as the proportion of the cardiac output that passes through unventilated alveoli (the shunt fraction) increases. It follows that the A–a gradient must increase with F_IO_2 and the shunt fraction (Figure 9.4B).

The PaO₂:F₁0₂ Ratio

An alternative method of assessing disease severity, and in particular the extent and severity of low $\dot{V}/\dot{Q}$ and unventilated alveoli, is to divide the PaO_2 by the F_IO_2. If, for example, a patient has a PaO_2 of 80 mmHg while receiving an F_IO_2 of 0.8, the PaO_2:F_IO_2 (or P:F) ratio is 80/0.8 or 100. The lower the P:F ratio, the more severe the disturbance in gas exchange. The P:F ratio is sometimes used in place of the A–a gradient as a measure of low $\dot{V}/\dot{Q}$ regions and shunt because it is thought (with little justification) to be less affected by changes in F_IO_2. It's also used to classify ARDS patients into those with mild, moderate, and severe disease (Chapter 12).

Venous Admixture and Shunt Fraction

The magnitude and severity of low $\dot{V}/\dot{Q}$ regions and shunt and their effect on gas exchange can also be assessed by calculating the *venous admixture* ($\dot{Q}_{VA}/\dot{Q}_T$). This calculation assumes that the lungs contain only ideal and non-ventilated alveoli (Figure 9.5). Recall from Chapter 2 that ideal alveoli have a $\dot{V}/\dot{Q}$ of approximately 1.0. The venous admixture is then the fraction of the mixed venous blood that would have to pass through non-ventilated alveoli to produce the calculated O_2 content (discussed later) of arterial blood. The venous admixture is equal to the difference between the O_2 content of ideal (CiO_2) and arterial (CaO_2) blood divided by the difference between the O_2 content of ideal and mixed venous ($C\overline{v}O_2$) blood. This is expressed mathematically as:

$$\dot{Q}_{VA}/\dot{Q}_T = \left(CiO_2 - CaO_2\right)/\left(CiO_2 - C\overline{v}O_2\right) \tag{9.4}$$

Alternatively, hemoglobin saturation can be substituted for oxygen content. If the saturation of ideal blood is assumed to be 100%, Equation 9.4 can be written as:

$$\dot{Q}_{VA}/\dot{Q}_T = \left(100 - SaO_2\right)/\left(100 - S\overline{v}O_2\right) \tag{9.5}$$

Here, $S\overline{v}O_2$ is the hemoglobin saturation of mixed venous blood.

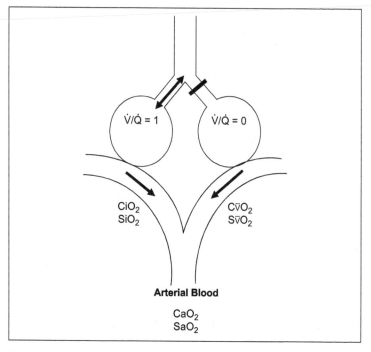

Figure 9.5 Calculation of the venous admixture is based on the assumption that the arterial blood oxygen content (CaO_2) and hemoglobin saturation (SaO_2) are the weighted average of the oxygen contents or hemoglobin saturations of the blood passing through "ideal" alveoli (CiO_2 and SiO_2) and unventilated alveoli ($C\bar{v}O_2$ and $S\bar{v}O_2$).

When F_iO_2 is 1.0, the blood leaving even very poorly ventilated alveoli has a hemoglobin saturation of 100%, so low $\dot{V}/\dot{Q}$ regions no longer contribute to the venous admixture. Equations 9.4 and 9.5 then allow us to calculate the fraction of the cardiac output that flows through intra-pulmonary and intra-cardiac right-to-left shunts, and this is referred to as the *shunt fraction* ($\dot{Q}_S/\dot{Q}_T$).

Physiologic Dead Space to Tidal Volume Ratio

From a conceptual standpoint, there are several parallels between the venous admixture and the dead space to tidal volume ratio. The venous admixture quantifies the effect of shunt and low $\dot{V}/\dot{Q}$ alveoli by assuming that the oxygen content or hemoglobin saturation of arterial blood is due to the mixing of blood from ideal alveoli with a fraction of the mixed venous blood. The ratio of physiologic dead space to tidal volume (V_D/V_T) quantifies the effect of high $\dot{V}/\dot{Q}$ and non-perfused alveoli plus the volume of the conducting airways by assuming that the PCO_2 of expired gas results from the mixing of gas leaving ideal alveoli with gas from non-perfused alveoli; i.e., inspired air (Figure 9.6). Figure 9.7 illustrates these similarities by modifying Figure 2.2 in Chapter 2 to show V_D/V_T and $\dot{Q}_{VA}/\dot{Q}_T$ as shunts that allow a portion of total ventilation and total perfusion to bypass the alveolar–capillary interface.

Analogous to $\dot{Q}_{VA}/\dot{Q}_T$, V_D/V_T is the difference between the PCO_2 of ideal alveolar gas ($PiCO_2$) and expired gas ($P\bar{E}CO_2$) divided by the difference between the PCO_2 of ideal alveolar gas and inspired gas. Since inspired gas can be assumed to have no CO_2, this can be expressed as:

$$V_D/V_T = \left(PiCO_2 - P\bar{E}CO_2\right)/PiCO_2 \tag{9.6}$$

The problem with Equation 9.6 is that $PiCO_2$ is a theoretical construct and cannot be measured. The Bohr-Enghoff equation, which substitutes $PaCO_2$ for $PiCO_2$, is most commonly used to overcome this problem.

$$V_D/V_T = \left(PaCO_2 - P\bar{E}CO_2\right)/PaCO_2 \tag{9.7}$$

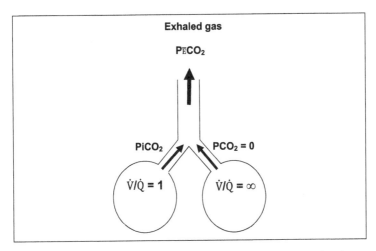

Figure 9.6 Calculation of the ratio of physiologic dead space to tidal volume is based on the assumption that the PCO_2 of mixed, expired gas ($P\bar{E}CO_2$) is the weighted average of the PCO_2 of gas leaving ideal alveoli ($PiCO_2$) and the PCO_2 of gas leaving unperfused alveoli.

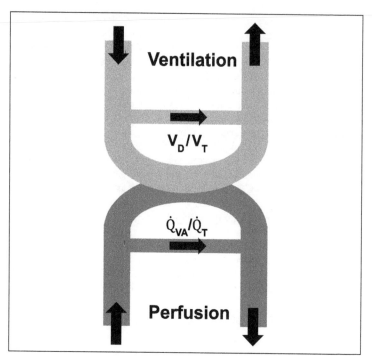

Figure 9.7 The venous admixture ($\dot{Q}_{VA}/\dot{Q}_T$) and the ratio of physiologic dead space to tidal volume (V_D/V_T) are depicted as shunts that allow a portion of the mixed venous blood and the inspired gas to bypass the alveolar gas–blood interface.

The mean PCO_2 of expired gas is usually measured using volume capnography, which will be discussed later in this chapter.

Recall from Chapter 2 that when V_D/V_T is low, alveolar volume is a large component of each breath, and ventilation is very effective at excreting CO_2 from the lungs. When V_D/V_T is high, most of each breath is dead space, and ventilation becomes very inefficient at removing CO_2.

Oxygen Content and Delivery

Recall from Chapter 2 that the oxygen content of arterial blood (CaO_2) is expressed as the volume of O_2 (in ml) carried by one deciliter (dl) of blood. If the very small volume of dissolved O_2 is neglected, arterial O_2 content is calculated as the product of the volume of O_2 carried by one gram (g) of fully saturated hemoglobin (1.34 ml/g), the hemoglobin concentration (Hb; g/dl), and the fractional arterial hemoglobin saturation ($SaO_2/100$).

$$CaO_2 = 1.34 \times Hb \times SaO_2 / 100 \qquad (9.8)$$

The volume of O_2 delivered by the arterial circulation (O_2 delivery; $\dot{D}O_2$) is calculated by multiplying CaO_2 by the cardiac output (CO).

$$\dot{D}O_2 = CaO_2 \times CO \times 10 \qquad (9.9)$$

Oxygen delivery is expressed as ml of oxygen/min, CO is in L/min, and multiplying by 10 converts CaO_2 from ml/dl to ml/L.

Arterial PCO_2

Also recall from Chapter 2 that $PaCO_2$ is determined by the balance between the rates at which CO_2 is produced by the body ($\dot{V}_PCO_2$) and excreted by the lungs ($\dot{V}_ECO_2$).

$$PaCO_2 \propto \dot{V}_PCO_2 / \dot{V}_ECO_2 \qquad (9.10)$$

CO_2 excretion is directly proportional to alveolar ventilation ($\dot{V}_A$), which is the volume of gas that moves into and out of optimally perfused alveoli each minute.

Since $\dot{V}_A$ is the difference between total (minute) ventilation ($\dot{V}_E$) and dead space ventilation ($\dot{V}_D$), Equation 9.11 can be rewritten as:

$$PaCO_2 \propto \dot{V}_PCO_2 / \dot{V}_E - \dot{V}_D \qquad (9.11)$$

This equation shows that measuring the $PaCO_2$ is a simple but very effective way to assess the adequacy of ventilation. An elevated $PaCO_2$ (hypercapnia) means that the respiratory system is unable to maintain the ventilation needed to excrete the CO_2 produced by the body, and this can be caused by a fall in $\dot{V}_E$, an increase in $\dot{V}_D$, or a rise in CO_2 production.

Hypocapnia (low $PaCO_2$) is caused by excessive alveolar ventilation. It often results from physical or psychological distress, but other common causes include metabolic acidosis, sepsis, and hepatic failure. As discussed in Chapter 8, hypocapnia in mechanically ventilated patients may also be iatrogenic and can be corrected by lowering the set mandatory rate.

Capnography

Capnography is the graphical display of the CO_2 content of respiratory gas. The partial pressure or fractional concentration (FCO_2) of carbon dioxide is measured using the same principle as co-oximetry and pulse oximetry. Gas between the endotracheal tube and the ventilator circuit is continuously exposed to infrared light at wavelengths absorbed by CO_2, and FCO_2 and PCO_2 are calculated by measuring the amount of absorbed and transmitted light. FCO_2, or more commonly, PCO_2 is displayed on the Y-axis and plotted against either time (*time capnography*) or exhaled volume (*volume capnography*). As shown in Figure 9.8, time-capnograms provide a continuous display throughout the entire respiratory cycle, whereas volume-capnograms show only expiration.

The exhaled portion of a time or volume-capnogram is conventionally divided into three phases (Figure 9.9). Phase I is due to emptying of the conducting airways. Since this gas didn't reach the alveoli during inspiration and didn't participate in gas exchange, it contains no CO_2, and PCO_2 is zero. During Phase II, PCO_2 increases rapidly as the remaining gas from the conducting airways mixes with an increasing volume of alveolar gas. Phase III

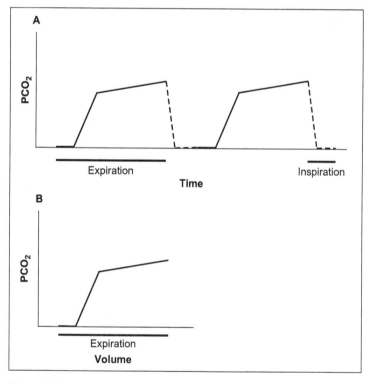

Figure 9.8 Time (A) and volume (B) capnograms. Expiration is shown by the solid line and inspiration by the dashed line.

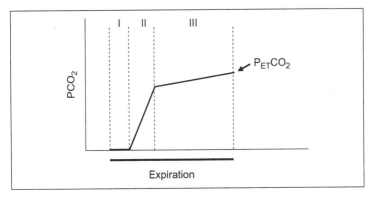

Figure 9.9 The three phases of expiration shown on a time or volume capnogram. The end-tidal PCO_2 ($P_{ET}CO_2$) is shown.

reflects the PCO_2 of pure alveolar gas; the normal, positive slope reflects the successive emptying of alveoli with worsening ventilation, falling $\dot{V}/\dot{Q}$, and increasing PCO_2. The PCO_2 at the end of expiration is called the *end-tidal* PCO_2 ($P_{ET}CO_2$).

Time Capnography

Time capnography is most often used to measure $P_{ET}CO_2$ as a noninvasive estimate of $PaCO_2$. Continuous monitoring of $P_{ET}CO_2$ has long been the standard of care in the operating room and is also commonly used to assure the adequacy of ventilation in patients receiving procedural sedation. The substitution of $P_{ET}CO_2$ for $PaCO_2$ is based on the assumption that the difference between these two measurements is small and fairly constant. In the absence of lung disease, this is generally true, and on average, $PaCO_2$ exceeds $P_{ET}CO_2$ by 3–6 mmHg.

In theory, $P_{ET}CO_2$ could also serve as a surrogate for $PaCO_2$ in mechanically ventilated ICU patients. This would be an attractive alternative to frequent blood gas measurements and could be used to adjust and monitor the effect of changes in ventilator settings. Unfortunately, studies have shown that the difference between $P_{ET}CO_2$ and $PaCO_2$ can vary widely and unpredictably in mechanically ventilated, critically ill patients. Even worse, $PaCO_2$ and $P_{ET}CO_2$ often move in opposite directions!

There are several reasons for this. First, alveolar dead space generated by high $\dot{V}/\dot{Q}$ and unperfused alveoli dilutes the expired PCO_2 and reduces $P_{ET}CO_2$ without changing $PaCO_2$. Second, intra-pulmonary shunting increases $PaCO_2$ without affecting $P_{ET}CO_2$.[1] Third, because Phase III has a positive slope,

1 The increase in respiratory drive and alveolar ventilation triggered by hypercapnia restores $PaCO_2$ to normal, but the accompanying dilution of the expired PCO_2 maintains the abnormal $PaCO_2$–$P_{ET}CO_2$ gradient.

$P_{ET}CO_2$ decreases when patients (especially those with obstructive lung disease) have insufficient time for complete exhalation. Finally, when cardiac output is reduced, the venous blood delivers less CO_2 to the lungs, less is excreted with each breath, and $P_{ET}CO_2$ falls. The bottom line is that $P_{ET}CO_2$ should not be used to estimate $PaCO_2$, or even to assess which direction it's moving in critically ill patients.

Volume Capnography

Volume capnography can also provide a continuous display of $P_{ET}CO_2$, but because it measures FCO_2 and PCO_2 relative to exhaled volume, it can also be used to perform a number of other measurements and calculations. This makes it much more useful than time capnography in the assessment and management of mechanically ventilated ICU patients.

CO_2 Excretion

The volume of CO_2 exhaled during a single breath ($VeCO_2$) is equal to the area under the FCO_2–volume curve (Figure 9.10). Multiplying $VeCO_2$ by the respiratory rate yields the volume of CO_2 excreted each minute ($\dot{V}eCO_2$).

Physiological Dead Space, Dead Space to Tidal Volume Ratio, Dead Space Ventilation, and Alveolar Ventilation

As previously discussed, V_D/V_T is calculated using the Bohr-Enghoff equation (Equation 9.7). $PaCO_2$ is measured from an arterial blood sample, and volume capnography is used to calculate the mean expired PCO_2 ($P\bar{E}CO_2$). This requires two steps. First, the mean expired fractional concentration of CO_2 ($F\bar{E}CO_2$) is determined by dividing the volume of expired CO_2 by the expired tidal volume.

$$F\bar{E}CO_2 = VeCO_2/V_T \tag{9.12}$$

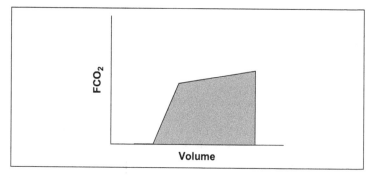

Figure 9.10 The volume of CO_2 exhaled with each breath is equal to the area under the plot of the fractional CO_2 concentration (FCO_2) versus expired volume.

Then, $F\bar{E}CO_2$ is multiplied by the total pressure of dry gas in the lungs; i.e., barometric pressure (P_B) minus the partial pressure of water (P_{H2O}).

$$P\bar{E}CO_2 = F\bar{E}CO_2 \times (P_B - P_{H2O})$$ (9.13)

Figure 9.11 shows the relationship between $PaCO_2$, $P_{ET}CO_2$, and $P\bar{E}CO_2$. Physiologic dead space (V_D) is calculated by multiplying V_D/V_T by the exhaled tidal volume, and multiplying by the respiratory rate gives dead space ventilation ($\dot{V}_D$). Alveolar ventilation ($\dot{V}_A$) is the difference between minute ventilation and dead space ventilation.

Airway and Alveolar Dead Space

Airway dead space (V_{D-AW}) is determined graphically by bisecting Phase II of the volume capnogram with a perpendicular line (Figure 9.12). This transforms Phase II from a gradual to an abrupt transition between airway and alveolar gas, and the volume to the left of the line is assumed to equal the airway dead space. Once physiologic and airway dead space have been determined, alveolar dead space (V_{D-ALV}) is calculated as the difference between them.

Fortunately, most modern volume capnographs perform all these measurements and calculations for you. All you have to do is measure and input the $PaCO_2$. The problem is figuring out practical and clinically relevant uses for all of this information. One promising application of volume capnography is to assist in identifying the appropriate level of PEEP in patients with the acute respiratory distress syndrome, and this will be discussed in Chapter 12.

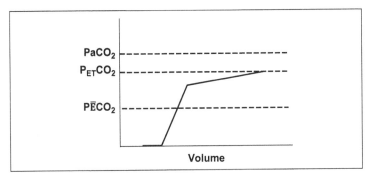

Figure 9.11 The arterial ($PaCO_2$), end-tidal ($P_{ET}CO_2$), and mean expired ($P\bar{E}CO_2$) are shown on this plot of PCO_2 versus expired volume.

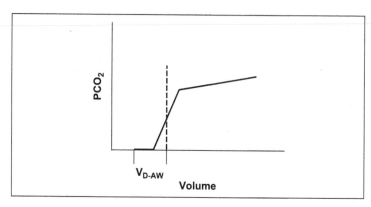

Figure 9.12 Airway dead space volume (V_{D-AW}) is equal to the volume to the left of a line that bisects Phase II of the volume capnogram.

Assessment of Respiratory Mechanics

Ventilation is possible only when the respiratory muscles or a mechanical ventilator provides enough pressure to overcome the elastic recoil and viscous forces of the respiratory system. Respiratory mechanics is the interaction of these applied and opposing forces and was discussed in detail in Chapter 1. Here, I focus on several clinically important measurements during a mechanical breath.

Airway and Alveolar Pressures

The *peak airway pressure* (P_{PEAK}) is the maximum airway pressure (P_{AW}) reached during a mechanical breath and can be read from the P_{AW}–time curve or the digital display on the ventilator user interface. During a passive, volume control (VC) breath with constant inspiratory flow, P_{AW} increases linearly with the delivered volume, and P_{PEAK} is reached at end-inspiration (Figure 9.13). During pressure control (PC), adaptive pressure control (aPC), pressure support (PS), and adaptive pressure support (aPS) breaths, P_{PEAK} equals the constant P_{AW} maintained throughout inspiration.

The *plateau pressure* (P_{PLAT}) is measured during an end-inspiratory pause, which holds the tidal volume in the lungs for a short time before expiration is allowed to proceed. Figure 9.13 shows the effect of an end-inspiratory pause during a passive VC breath. Since there are no viscous forces in the absence of flow, P_{PLAT} is the end-inspiratory alveolar pressure (P_{ALV}). It is also the sum of the pressure needed to balance the increase in elastic recoil during inspiration (P_{ER}) and total PEEP ($PEEP_T$). Like P_{PEAK}, P_{PLAT} can be read from either the graphical or the digital display on the user interface.

Total PEEP ($PEEP_T$) is the sum of set or extrinsic PEEP ($PEEP_E$) and intrinsic PEEP ($PEEP_I$) due to dynamic hyperinflation. Total PEEP equals end-expiratory

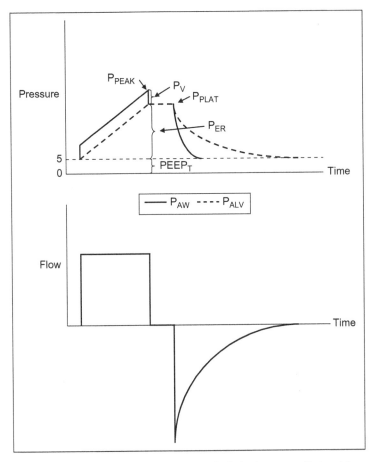

Figure 9.13 Simultaneous plots of airway pressure (P_{AW}), alveolar pressure (P_{ALV}), and flow vs. time during a passive, volume control breath with constant inspiratory flow and a brief end-inspiratory pause. Total PEEP ($PEEP_T$) of 5 cmH$_2$O is present. During the end-inspiratory pause, peak airway pressure (P_{PEAK}) rapidly falls to plateau pressure (P_{PLAT}), which equals alveolar pressure at end-inspiration and the total elastic recoil pressure of the respiratory system. The difference between P_{PLAT} and $PEEP_T$ is the pressure needed to balance the elastic recoil generated by the tidal volume (P_{ER}). The difference between P_{PEAK} and P_{PLAT} is the pressure needed to overcome viscous forces (P_V) just before the end-inspiratory pause.

P_{ALV}, which is the total elastic recoil pressure of the respiratory system just before the next mechanical breath. As shown in Figure 9.13, P_{ALV} and flow decrease exponentially during expiration, and flow stops only when P_{ALV} has returned to zero (atmospheric pressure) or to the level of $PEEP_E$.

Notice that P_{AW} reaches this pressure well before P_{ALV} does. You can understand why by looking at Figure 9.14. Mechanical ventilators measure P_{AW}

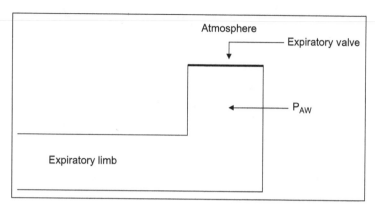

Figure 9.14 Schematic diagram showing the site of airway pressure (P_{AW}) measurement relative to the expiratory valve.

proximal to the expiratory valve. Throughout inspiration, the expiratory valve is closed, so P_{AW} equals the pressure in the ventilator circuit and the large airways of the lungs. During expiration, though, the expiratory valve opens and the pressure sensor is exposed to $PEEP_E$. That's why P_{AW} falls so quickly and why it doesn't reflect P_{ALV} during expiration.

$PEEP_T$ can be measured during an end-expiratory pause, which closes the expiratory valve and stops any remaining expiratory flow. As shown in Figure 9.15,

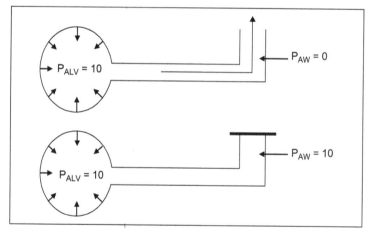

Figure 9.15 Schematic diagram showing that closing the expiratory valve allows pressure to equalize throughout the circuit so that airway pressure (P_{AW}) equals alveolar pressure (P_{ALV}), which equals total PEEP.

this allows pressure to equilibrate between the lungs and the ventilator circuit, and P_{AW} becomes equal to P_{ALV}. If expiratory flow has already stopped and the respiratory system has reached its equilibrium position, $PEEP_T$ will equal $PEEP_E$. When expiratory time is insufficient to allow complete exhalation, $PEEP_T$ will equal the sum of $PEEP_E$ and $PEEP_I$ (Figure 9.16). Chapter 10 is devoted to dynamic hyperinflation and $PEEP_I$.

Before performing an end-expiratory pause, you can "screen" for $PEEP_I$ simply by looking at the expiratory flow–time curve. As shown in Figure 9.17, if expiratory flow stops before the onset of the next mechanical breath, $PEEP_T$ must equal $PEEP_E$. If end-expiratory flow is greater than zero, $PEEP_I$ must be present, and $PEEP_T$ will exceed $PEEP_E$.

Compliance and Resistance

Remember from Chapter 1 that elastic recoil is most often expressed in terms of *compliance* (C), which is the ratio of the volume change (ΔV) produced by a change in transmural pressure (ΔP_{TM}).

$$C = \Delta V / \Delta P_{TM} \tag{9.14}$$

Viscous forces are quantified by *resistance* (R), which is the intramural pressure gradient between two points of a tube or circuit (ΔP_{IM}) divided by the flow that it produces ($\dot{V}$).

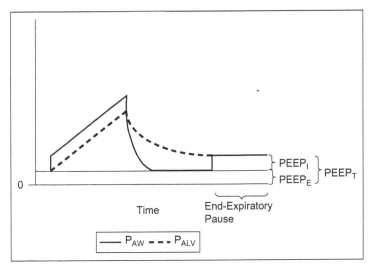

Figure 9.16 During expiration, P_{AW} rapidly falls to the set level of PEEP ($PEEP_E$). When an end-expiratory pause is performed, P_{AW} equals P_{ALV} and total PEEP ($PEEP_T$), and the difference between $PEEP_T$ and extrinsic PEEP is intrinsic PEEP ($PEEP_I$).

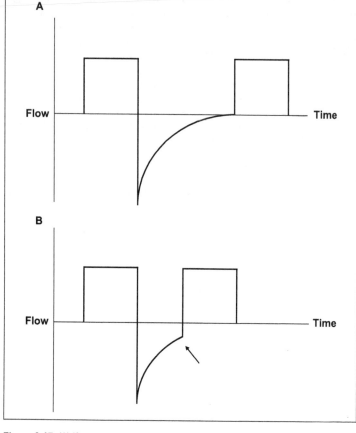

Figure 9.17 (A) If expiratory flow reaches zero before the next mechanical breath, PEEP$_T$ will equal PEEP$_E$, and PEEP$_I$ will be zero.

(B) If expiratory flow persists at end-expiration (*arrow*), PEEP$_I$ must be present, and PEEP$_T$ will exceed PEEP$_E$.

$$R = \Delta P_{IM} / \dot{V} \qquad (9.15)$$

Both the compliance and resistance of the respiratory system can be calculated from measurements obtained during a passive, VC breath (Figure 9.13). Respiratory system compliance (C$_{RS}$) over the tidal volume range is equal to the set tidal volume (V$_T$) divided by the pressure needed to overcome elastic recoil (P_{ER}), which is the difference between P_{ALV} at the end of inspiration (P_{PLAT}) and the end of expiration ($PEEP_T$).

$$C_{RS} = V_T / (P_{PLAT} - PEEP_T) \tag{9.16}$$

Respiratory system resistance (R_{RS}) is equal to the pressure needed to overcome viscous forces (P_V) divided by the end-inspiratory flow rate ($\dot{V}_{EI}$). Since viscous forces disappear during an end-inspiratory pause, P_V is the difference between P_{PEAK} and P_{PLAT}.

$$R_{RS} = (P_{PEAK} - P_{PLAT}) / \dot{V}_{EI} \tag{9.17}$$

Although compliance and resistance calculations are fairly straightforward, there are several things to keep in mind. First, V_T and end-inspiratory flow must be known. That's why you must use a volume-control breath with a set, constant inspiratory flow rate. Second, the measured P_{PEAK}, P_{PLAT}, and $PEEP_T$ will be accurate only if ventilation is passive. Patient effort can usually be minimized by providing sufficient sedation. Alternatively, you can induce hypocapnia by briefly increasing the set respiratory rate. This will reduce the patient's respiratory drive, and when the rate is decreased, a brief period of apnea will usually allow accurate pressure measurements to be obtained.

Additional Reading

Bekos V, Marini JJ. Monitoring the mechanically-ventilated patient. *Crit Care Clin.* 2007;23:575–611.

Hess DR. Respiratory mechanics in mechanically ventilated patients. *Respir Care.* 2014;59:1773–1794.

Truwitt JD, Marini JJ. Evaluation of thoracic mechanics in the ventilated patient. Part 1: primary measurements. *J Crit Care.* 1988;3:133–150.

Truwitt JD, Marini JJ. Evaluation of thoracic mechanics in the ventilated patient. Part 2: applied mechanics. *J Crit Care.* 1988;3:199–213.

Chapter 10

Dynamic Hyperinflation and Intrinsic Positive End-Expiratory Pressure

Normally, expiratory flow stops and expiration ends only when the respiratory system has returned to its equilibrium volume and alveolar pressure (P_{ALV}) is zero (Figure 10.1A). This is the point at which the elastic recoil of the lungs and the chest wall are equal and opposite (see Chapter 1). Clinician-added or "extrinsic" positive end-expiratory pressure ($PEEP_E$) creates a new, higher equilibrium volume, and end-expiratory alveolar pressure (P_{ALVee}) equals $PEEP_E$ (Figure 10.1B).

When the time available for expiration (expiratory time; T_E) is insufficient to allow the respiratory system to return to its equilibrium volume with or without $PEEP_E$ (Figure 10.2), flow persists at end-expiration, and P_{ALVee} exceeds $PEEP_E$ by an amount referred to as *intrinsic PEEP* ($PEEP_I$). P_{ALVee} is then the sum of extrinsic and intrinsic PEEP, which is called *total PEEP* ($PEEP_T$).

$$P_{ALVee} = PEEP_T = (PEEP_E + PEEP_I) \tag{10.1}$$

Intrinsic PEEP (or auto-PEEP) results from *dynamic hyperinflation,* which is illustrated in Figure 10.3. When T_E is too short to allow the entire tidal volume (V_T) to be exhaled, there is a progressive increase in lung volume. The accompanying rise in elastic recoil increases expiratory flow, which eventually allows a relatively constant end-inspiratory and end-expiratory lung volume (and $PEEP_I$) to be established.

Dynamic hyperinflation and $PEEP_I$ almost always occur in patients with severe obstructive lung disease, in whom slowing of expiratory flow prevents complete exhalation even when T_E is normal or prolonged. Occasionally, patients without airflow obstruction develop dynamic hyperinflation when T_E is excessively shortened by a rapid respiratory rate, a long set inspiratory time (T_I), or both.

Diagnosis of Dynamic Hyperinflation and Intrinsic PEEP

Clinical Indicators

Dynamic hyperinflation should always be suspected in mechanically ventilated patients with obstructive lung disease. The presence of breath sounds or

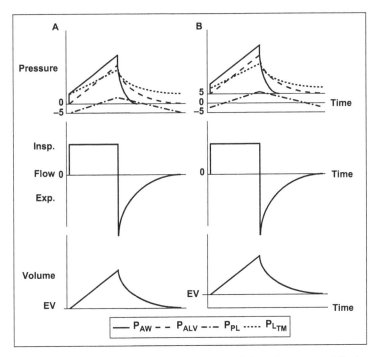

Figure 10.1 Plots of airway (P_{AW}), alveolar (P_{ALV}), pleural (P_{PL}), and lung transmural (P_{LTM}) pressure, flow, and volume during a respiratory cycle with $PEEP_E$ of zero (A) and 5 cmH$_2$O (B). $PEEP_E$ creates a higher equilibrium volume (EV) and increases P_{AW}, P_{ALV}, P_{PL}, P_{LTM}, and end-inspiratory and end-expiratory lung volume. Alveolar pressure at end-expiration equals $PEEP_E$.

wheezing that continues throughout the entire expiratory phase is the most suggestive sign, although its absence certainly does not exclude the diagnosis. Dynamic hyperinflation must also be strongly suspected when patients develop one or more characteristic complications, specifically hypotension and ineffective ventilator triggering (discussed later in this chapter).

Qualitative Measures

As discussed in Chapter 9, you can screen for $PEEP_I$ by examining the flow–time curve on the user interface (Figure 10.2). If expiratory flow doesn't reach zero before the next mechanical breath, dynamic hyperinflation must be present. The higher the end-expiratory flow, the more severe the dynamic hyperinflation, and the greater the $PEEP_I$.

Quantitative Measures

$PEEP_T$ and $PEEP_I$ can be measured during a brief end-expiratory pause (Chapter 9). Remember that the ventilator measures airway pressure (P_{AW})

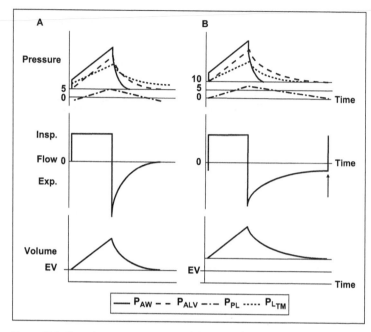

Figure 10.2 Plots of airway (P_{AW}), alveolar (P_{ALV}), pleural (P_{PL}), and lung transmural ($P_{L_{TM}}$) pressure, flow, and volume with PEEP$_E$ of 5 cmH$_2$O and PEEP$_I$ of zero (A) and 5 cmH$_2$O (B). PEEP$_I$ occurs when there is insufficient time for complete exhalation. This is indicated by persistent flow at end-expiration (*arrow*). PEEP$_I$ further increases P_{AW}, P_{ALV}, P_{PL}, $P_{L_{TM}}$, and end-inspiratory and end-expiratory lung volume. Alveolar pressure at end-expiration equals the sum of PEEP$_E$ and PEEP$_I$. EV is the equilibrium volume produced by PEEP$_E$.

proximal to the expiratory valve. Throughout expiration, when the expiratory valve is open, P_{AW} equals zero (atmospheric pressure) or the set level of PEEP$_E$, not P_{ALV}. When the valve is closed during an end-expiratory pause, flow stops, pressure equilibrates between the alveoli and the pressure sensor,

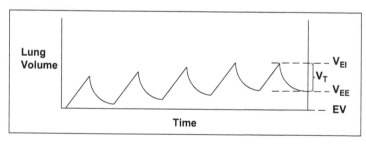

Figure 10.3 When there is insufficient time to exhale the delivered tidal volume (V_T), end-inspiratory (V_{EI}) and end-expiratory (V_{EE}) volume increase above the equilibrium volume of the respiratory system (EV) until a plateau is reached.

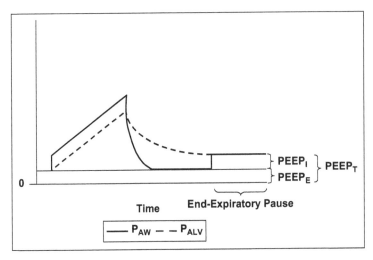

Figure 10.4 Airway pressure (P_{AW}) and alveolar pressure (P_{ALV}) vs. time in a patient with dynamic hyperinflation. During an end-expiratory pause, P_{AW} rapidly increases to reach P_{ALV}, which equals total PEEP ($PEEP_T$). Intrinsic PEEP ($PEEP_I$) is the difference between $PEEP_T$ and extrinsic PEEP ($PEEP_E$).

and P_{AW} equals P_{ALVee} ($PEEP_T$) (Figure 10.4). $PEEP_I$ can then be calculated as the difference between $PEEP_T$ and $PEEP_E$.

Also recall that the measurements performed during an end-expiratory pause will be accurate only if the patient is not attempting to breathe. Often, sedation will sufficiently minimize patient effort. Alternatively, accurate pressure measurements can usually be obtained once respiratory drive has been decreased by a brief period of hyperventilation.

As shown in Figure 10.5, dynamic hyperinflation can be directly quantified by stopping ventilation in a pharmacologically paralyzed patient and measuring expired volume until flow reaches zero. The volume of the expired gas is the difference between end-inspiratory volume (V_{EI}) and the equilibrium volume (EV) of the respiratory system. The difference between end-expiratory volume (V_{EE}) and EV can then be determined by subtracting the tidal volume. Since it provides little clinically useful information and requires neuromuscular blockade, this measurement is typically restricted to research studies.

Consequences of Dynamic Hyperinflation

Dynamic hyperinflation can cause three important adverse effects in mechanically ventilated patients.

- Reduced cardiac output and hypotension
- Barotrauma
- Ineffective ventilator triggering

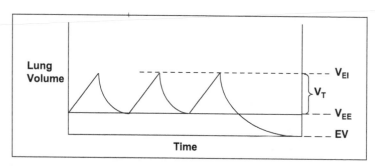

Figure 10.5 A pharmacologically paralyzed patient with dynamic hyperinflation will reach the equilibrium volume of the respiratory system (EV) during a period of apnea. The exhaled volume is the difference between end-inspiratory volume (V_{EI}) and EV. The difference between end-expiratory volume (V_{EE}) and EV is determined by subtracting the tidal volume (V_T).

Reduced Cardiac Output and Hypotension

As discussed in Chapter 3 and shown in Figure 10.1A, mechanical ventilation causes a *cyclical* increase in pleural (P_{PL}) and lung transmural (PL_{TM}) pressure. By increasing end-expiratory lung volume, both $PEEP_E$ and $PEEP_I$ cause an additional, *continuous* rise in P_{PL} and PL_{TM} (Figures 10.1B and 10.2), which leads to further reduction in venous return and further increase in RV afterload, respectively. If sufficiently large, the decrease in preload and increase in afterload will cause cardiac output and blood pressure to fall.

Barotrauma

By increasing lung volume throughout the respiratory cycle (Figures 10.2B and 10.3), dynamic hyperinflation predisposes to alveolar over-distension, and this may lead to alveolar rupture, which is usually referred to as "barotrauma." Air tracks along the bronchovascular bundles and enters the mediastinum (pneumomediastinum). From there, air may enter the pleural space (pneumothorax), the subcutaneous tissues (subcutaneous emphysema), and even the pericardial space (pneumopericardium) or the abdominal compartment (pneumoperitoneum). Pneumothorax interferes with gas exchange and may cause hypotension by further increasing P_{PL} and reducing venous return. Pneumopericardium may impair cardiac filling and cause cardiac tamponade.

Ineffective Ventilator Triggering

Consider what must occur before a patient with dynamic hyperinflation can trigger a mechanical breath (Figure 10.6). During expiration, the respiratory system is above its equilibrium volume, inward elastic recoil raises P_{ALV} above the pressure at the expiratory valve (P_{AW}), and gas flows from the lungs (Figure 10.6A). P_{AW} is equal to $PEEP_E$. If the patient attempts to trigger

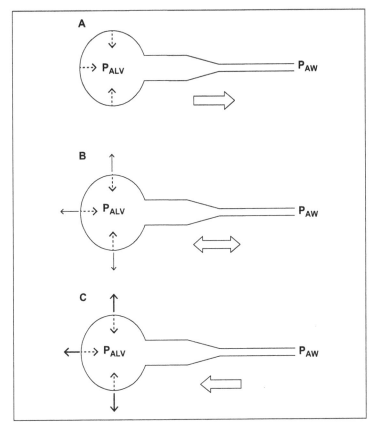

Figure 10.6 Schematic diagrams showing the steps necessary for a patient with dynamic hyperinflation to trigger a mechanical breath.

(A) Just before an inspiratory effort, the inward elastic recoil (*dashed arrows*) produces the gradient between alveolar pressure (P_{ALV}) and airway pressure (P_{AW}), and gas flows from the lungs (*large, open arrow*).

(B) In order to stop expiratory flow (*large, double-sided open arrow*), the patient must reduce P_{ALV} until it equals P_{AW} ($PEEP_E$), and this requires a pressure equal to $PEEP_I$ (*solid, thin arrows*).

(C) To trigger a mechanical breath (*large, open arrow*), the patient must then lower P_{ALV} even further (*solid, thick arrows*) to reduce P_{AW} or the base flow.

a breath before P_{ALV} has reached $PEEP_E$, they must first stop expiratory flow. This can be done only by generating enough inspiratory pressure to eliminate the pressure gradient that is driving flow. That is, they must lower P_{ALV} until it reaches $PEEP_E$ (Figure 10.6B). Since P_{ALV} equals $PEEP_T$, this requires a pressure equal to $PEEP_I$. Once expiratory flow stops, additional muscular effort is needed to trigger the ventilator (Figure 10.6C). As discussed in Chapter 4, if pressure triggering is used, P_{ALV} must be reduced enough to lower P_{AW} by the set sensitivity. If the ventilator is set for flow triggering, P_{ALV} must be decreased until the base flow falls by the set flow sensitivity.

Let's look at some examples to help clarify these concepts. If $PEEP_I$ is 10 cmH$_2$O, $PEEP_E$ is 0 cmH$_2$O ($PEEP_T$ = 10 cmH$_2$O), and the set pressure sensitivity is −2 cmH$_2$O, a patient must first lower P_{ALV} from 10 cmH$_2$O to zero and then generate an additional 2 cmH$_2$O to trigger the ventilator (total of 12 cmH$_2$O). If $PEEP_E$ and $PEEP_I$ are both 5 cmH$_2$O ($PEEP_T$ = 10 cmH$_2$O), P_{ALV} must be reduced from 10 cmH$_2$O to 5 cmH$_2$O to stop expiratory flow, and an additional 2 cmH$_2$O is needed to trigger the ventilator (total of 7 cmH$_2$O).

By forcing patients to stop expiratory flow before they can take another breath, dynamic hyperinflation produces a *threshold load* on the inspiratory muscles. Dynamic hyperinflation also forces patients to breathe at a higher, less compliant portion of the pressure–volume curve (see Chapter 1, Figure 1.3). Take a deep breath and then perform tidal breathing near total lung capacity. You'll discover that it's very difficult and very uncomfortable, and you'll be able to better appreciate the effort required to sustain ventilation.

Ineffective triggering occurs when a patient is unable to generate the inspiratory pressure needed to trigger the ventilator. This can usually be detected at the bedside by noting chest wall expansion and accessory muscle activity that do not trigger a mechanical breath. As shown in Figure 10.7, airway pressure and flow tracings may also reveal ineffective inspiratory efforts. Ineffective triggering will be discussed again in Chapter 11.

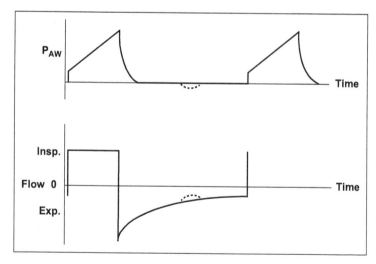

Figure 10.7 Ineffective triggering may cause deflections (*dotted lines*) on the airway pressure (P_{AW})–time and flow–time curves.

Management of Dynamic Hyperinflation

There are two ways to reduce the adverse effects of dynamic hyperinflation. The first is to decrease dynamic hyperinflation itself by allowing the respiratory system to get closer to its equilibrium volume. The second is to treat the adverse hemodynamic effects of $PEEP_I$.

Reducing Dynamic Hyperinflation

Since patients almost always have significant obstructive lung disease, bronchodilators and steroids may increase expiratory flow and reduce end-expiratory volume. At the same time, three ventilator adjustments can be made to allow more complete exhalation.

- Decrease the set respiratory rate (RR). If the patient is making no spontaneous efforts, this will reduce the total rate and increase the time between breaths, which will allow more complete emptying.
- Decrease the tidal volume (V_T). Since less volume is delivered, less must be exhaled, and the respiratory system will get closer to its equilibrium volume. With VC and aPC breaths, this is done by changing the set V_T. With PC breaths, V_T is reduced by lowering the driving pressure.
- Reduce inspiratory time (T_I). If respiratory cycle duration ($T_I + T_E$) is unchanged, a decrease in T_I must lengthen T_E, and this will reduce end-expiratory volume. Depending on the ventilator and the type of mechanical breath, inspiratory time can be decreased either by changing the set T_I or by increasing the set inspiratory flow rate.

It's important to recognize several important limitations of these ventilator adjustments.

First, inspiratory time is almost always very short to begin with, so decreasing it further does little to reduce dynamic hyperinflation. Let's say that a patient has a respiratory rate of 12. This means that every respiratory cycle lasts for $60/12 = 5$ seconds. If T_I is initially 1 second, T_E will be 4 seconds. If you reduce T_I to 0.5 second, T_E increases only to 4.5 seconds, and this is likely to have no clinically significant effect on $PEEP_I$.

Second, when attempting to reduce RR, V_T, or both, you will often encounter two problems. First, decreasing the set rate will have no effect if the patient is triggering additional mechanical breaths. Second, reducing V_T will not be beneficial if the patient increases their respiratory rate to compensate for the drop in minute ventilation.

Because of these limitations, patients with dynamic hyperinflation-induced hypotension who are unresponsive to volume expansion (see next section) may require sedation and neuromuscular blockade to allow sufficient reduction in RR or V_T to reduce $PEEP_I$. This usually leads to significant hypercapnia and respiratory acidosis, which can be treated, if necessary, with intravenous (IV) sodium bicarbonate.

Reducing Adverse Hemodynamic Effects

Intravenous Fluids

Since PEEP$_i$-induced hypotension is caused largely by a decrease in venous return, it can be treated by rapidly expanding intravascular volume. As discussed in detail in Chapter 3, this raises systemic venous pressure, increases the gradient driving blood into the RA, and improves RV and LV preload. Typically, 500 ml boluses of normal saline or Lactated Ringers are given until hypotension resolves or no further effect is seen.

Additional Reading

Blanch L, Bernabe F, Lucangelo U. Measurement of air trapping, intrinsic positive end-expiratory pressure, and dynamic hyperinflation in mechanically ventilated patients. *Respir Care*. 2005;50:110–123.

Calverley PM, Koulouris NG. Flow limitation and dynamic hyperinflation: Key concepts in modern respiratory physiology. *Eur Respir J*. 2005;25:186–199.

Dhand R. Ventilator graphics and respiratory mechanics in the patient with obstructive lung disease. *Respir Care*. 2005;50:246–261.

Pepe PE, Marini JJ. Occult positive end-expiratory pressure in mechanically ventilated patients with airflow obstruction. *Am Rev Respir Dis*. 1982;126:166–170.

Patient–Ventilator Interactions and Asynchrony

Effective mechanical ventilation requires the synchronized function of two pumps. One pump, the mechanical ventilator, is governed by the settings chosen by the clinician. The other, the patient's respiratory system, is controlled by groups of neurons in the brain stem that set the respiratory rate, inspiratory flow rate, and tidal volume based on input from peripheral and central chemoreceptors, intrapulmonary receptors, and the cerebral cortex. Ideally, these two pumps should work together so that the ventilator simply augments and amplifies the activity of the respiratory system. This is important because asynchrony between the ventilator and the patient reduces patient comfort, increases the work of breathing, predisposes the patient to respiratory muscle fatigue, and may even impair oxygenation and ventilation.

Patient–ventilator asynchrony most commonly occurs either during ventilator triggering or during the inspiratory phase of the respiratory cycle. This chapter explains how to detect asynchrony and describes how to reduce or eliminate it.

Asynchrony During Triggering

A mechanical breath is triggered when patient inspiratory effort causes the demand valve to open, which allows gas to flow into the lungs. As described in Chapter 4, the ventilator senses patient effort by detecting changes in either pressure or flow within the ventilator circuit. Three signs of patient–ventilator asynchrony may be evident during the triggering phase of a mechanical breath:

- Ineffective triggering
- Auto-triggering
- Multiple triggering

Ineffective Triggering

As the name indicates, ineffective triggering occurs when patient inspiratory effort is insufficient to trigger a mechanical breath. This can be detected in two ways. First, examine the patient while listening to the ventilator and look for any uncoupling of respiratory effort and mechanical breaths. Inspiratory efforts can be subtle and may be visible only as retractions just above the suprasternal notch. If the patient makes an inspiratory effort but does not receive a mechanical breath, triggering is ineffective. Second, look at the pressure–time curve on the ventilator user interface. As shown in Figure 11.1, patient inspiratory effort may be (but is not always) reflected by a drop in P_{AW} during the expiratory phase. The absence of an accompanying mechanical breath is diagnostic of ineffective triggering.

Ineffective triggering has three causes:

- Poor inspiratory effort (usually due to over-sedation)
- An inappropriately low (i.e., insensitive) trigger sensitivity
- Inability to overcome the "threshold load" produced by intrinsic PEEP ($PEEP_I$)

The last cause is by far the most common. Recall from Chapter 10 that when the respiratory system is above its equilibrium volume, a patient trying to trigger a mechanical breath must first stop expiratory flow by generating pressure equal to $PEEP_I$. Additional pressure must then be supplied to lower P_{AW} or the base flow sufficiently to trigger a mechanical breath.

When ineffective triggering is present, its cause must be identified and, if possible, corrected. The recognition and management of dynamic hyperinflation and $PEEP_I$ was discussed in Chapters 9 and 10, and I'll only emphasize a few points here.

- You can screen for dynamic hyperinflation by examining the flow–time curve on the user interface. As shown in Chapter 9, Figure 9.17, $PEEP_I$ must be present if expiratory flow does not return to zero prior to the next mechanical breath. $PEEP_I$ can then be quantified by measuring P_{AW} during a brief end-expiratory pause (Figure 9.16).
- Remember that $PEEP_I$ usually occurs in the setting of significant obstructive lung disease when the interval between mechanical breaths is insufficient to allow the respiratory system to return to its equilibrium volume. Intrinsic PEEP can most effectively be reduced by decreasing tidal volume, respiratory rate, or both.

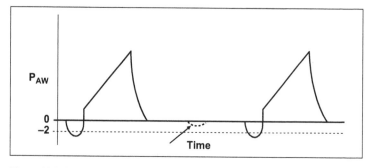

Figure 11.1 Patient inspiratory effort that is insufficient to trigger a breath may appear as a deflection (*dotted lines and arrow*) on the airway pressure (P_{AW})–time curve.

When PEEP$_I$ is not present, ineffective triggering can usually be corrected by reducing sedation or by increasing trigger sensitivity.

Auto-Triggering

Auto-triggering occurs when the ventilator initiates mechanical breaths in response to a drop in pressure or flow that is not produced by patient effort. Occasionally, this is caused by the back and forth movement of water in the ventilator circuit or by the heartbeat of a patient with a wide pulse pressure. More often, the drop in P$_{AW}$ or base flow is caused by a leak in the ventilator circuit. This may occur at a tubing connection or result from gas escaping around the cuff of the endotracheal or tracheostomy tube.

How does a leak cause auto-triggering? Remember that flow-triggering occurs whenever flow passing through the expiratory limb of the ventilator circuit falls below the base flow by a set amount (the flow-sensitivity). This, of course, usually means that the patient has started to inhale. But you can see that triggering will be independent of patient effort if there is a big enough leak in the ventilator circuit. Similarly, during pressure-triggering, a breath will be initiated if a leak causes a sufficient drop in P$_{AW}$. Unlike flow-triggering though, this will happen only if expiratory P$_{AW}$ is positive; that is, if extrinsic PEEP (PEEP$_E$) is present. That's because a leak can decrease P$_{AW}$ only if it's above atmospheric pressure. For example, if PEEP$_E$ is 5 cmH$_2$O and pressure sensitivity is set at -2 cmH$_2$O, a leak will trigger a mechanical breath when P$_{AW}$ drops below 3 cmH$_2$O. If PEEP$_E$ is zero, there's no way that P$_{AW}$ can fall below atmospheric pressure to -2 cmH$_2$O without patient inspiratory effort.

Not uncommonly, none of these causes is evident, and auto-triggering is due simply to an inappropriately high sensitivity (i.e., very sensitive) setting. This is particularly likely during flow-triggering when the sensitivity is set at or below 1 L/min.

Auto-triggering should be suspected in any patient who has a persistent and unexplained respiratory alkalosis. Like ineffective triggering, the diagnosis can usually be made by simultaneously looking at the patient and listening to the ventilator. In most cases, it's fairly obvious that mechanical breaths are not preceded by patient inspiratory effort.

Once auto-triggering has been confirmed, attention must be directed to identifying and correcting the cause. Make sure that flow-sensitivity has been set above 1 L/min. Carefully examine the ventilator circuit for leaks and drain any water that's present. Auscultate over the neck to detect air escaping around the cuff of the endotracheal or tracheostomy tube.

If the cause of auto-triggering remains unclear, it's probably due to an unrecognized leak, so here's what you do to confirm it. First, if the ventilator is set for flow-triggering, change it to pressure-triggering. Sometimes this, by itself, will eliminate the problem. If auto-triggering persists, reduce PEEP$_E$ to zero (if this is safe to do). For the reasons discussed previously, if auto-triggering stops, it must have been due to a leak, and additional efforts must be made to identify the source.

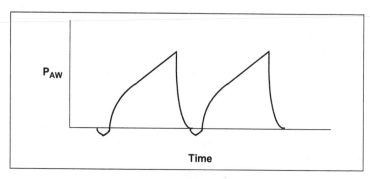

Figure 11.2 Multiple triggering indicates that the delivered tidal volume does not meet the needs of the patient.

Multiple Triggering

This type of patient–ventilator asynchrony occurs when a single inspiratory effort triggers several (usually two) mechanical breaths in rapid succession (Figure 11.2). When you see multiple triggering, it almost always means that the patient wants a much larger tidal volume. This causes the patient to continue to inhale after the ventilator cycles, which immediately triggers another mechanical breath. Multiple triggering can usually be minimized or eliminated by increasing the delivered tidal volume. When low tidal volume ventilation is needed for a patient with ARDS, increased sedation is often the only way to improve patient comfort and reduce patient–ventilator asynchrony.

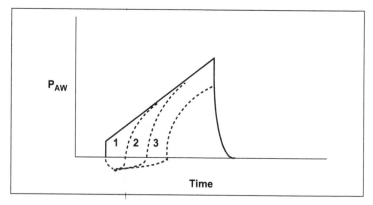

Figure 11.3 The more the patient's flow requirements exceed the set flow rate of a volume control breath (1 → 2 → 3), the greater the alteration of the airway pressure (P_{AW}) – time curve.

Asynchrony During Inspiration

Two signs of patient–ventilator asynchrony during inspiration are:

• Abnormally low airway pressure
• A spike in airway pressure at end-inspiration

Abnormally Low Airway Pressure

This occurs primarily with VC breaths and is a sign of inadequate inspiratory flow. Recall from Chapter 5 that inspiratory flow during VC breaths cannot be increased by patient effort. Patients who are dyspneic and tachypneic pull vigorously in an unsuccessful attempt to inflate their lungs more rapidly. Since the ventilator circuit is a closed system, when a patient inhales faster than gas enters the lungs, P_{AW} must fall, and this causes the P_{AW}–time curve to have a characteristic "scooped out" appearance. As shown in Figure 11.3, the degree and duration of the P_{AW} drop correlate with the magnitude of the imbalance between the set inspiratory flow and the demands of the patient. Notice that peak airway pressure (P_{PEAK}) often falls as this imbalance worsens.

The solution to this problem, of course, is to increase the inspiratory flow rate. At the same time, an effort should be made to identify and, if possible, correct the problem(s) leading to tachypnea and high flow requirements. Common causes include pain, anxiety, sepsis, and metabolic acidosis. Alternatively, you can switch from volume control to adaptive pressure control (aPC) breaths. But be careful. Even though aPC breaths are better able to match inspiratory flow demands, the ventilator provides less and less support

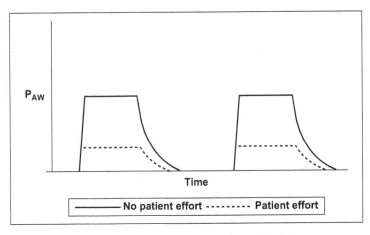

Figure 11.4 Plots of airway pressure (P_{AW}) versus time showing that the inspiratory pressure provided during adaptive pressure control breaths decreases as patient effort increases.

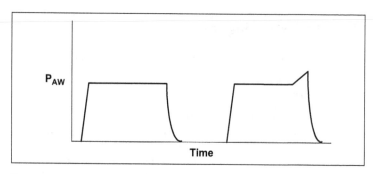

Figure 11.5 Patient exhalation during mechanical inflation causes an abrupt rise in airway pressure (P_{AW}).

as patient effort increases. This is reflected by a relatively small increase in airway pressure during inspiration and indicates that the patient is doing much or even most of the work of breathing (Figure 11.4).

End-Inspiratory Pressure Spike

When inspiratory time (T_I) is too long, the patient tries to exhale before mechanical inflation ends. Simultaneous, oppositely-directed flow from the ventilator and the patient causes an abrupt rise in P_{AW}, which can be detected by looking at the P_{AW}–time curve on the user interface (Figure 11.5). This is also a common cause of a high airway pressure alarm (see Chapter 6). When this problem is identified, T_I can be reduced either directly or by increasing the set flow rate, depending on the breath type and the ventilator being used (see Chapter 5).

Additional Reading

Georgopoulos D, Prinianakis G, Kondili E. Bedside waveforms interpretation as a tool to identify patient–ventilator asynchronies. *Intensive Care Med*. 2006;32:34–47.

Murias G, Villagra A, Blanch L. Patient–ventilator dyssynchrony during assisted invasive mechanical ventilation. *Minerva Anestesiol*. 2013;79:434–444.

Nilsestuen JO, Hargett KD. Using ventilator graphics to identify patient–ventilator asynchrony. *Respir Care*. 2005;50:202–234.

Chapter 12

Acute Respiratory Distress Syndrome (ARDS)

Definition

ARDS is a syndrome. In order to study its epidemiology and clinical course and enroll appropriate patients in clinical trials, it is essential to have a validated and widely accepted definition. During the past 50 years, as we have learned more about ARDS, its defining characteristics have been modified several times. In 2011, an international panel of experts convened in Berlin, Germany, in an attempt to more accurately define the syndrome and stratify its severity. After likely spending several months trying to come up with just the right name, the *Berlin Definition* of ARDS was published in 2012 (Table 12.1).

The consensus conference also defined three levels of severity based on the PaO_2/F_IO_2 (P/F) ratio (Table 12.2).

Table 12.1 The Berlin Definition of the Acute Respiratory Distress Syndrome	
Timing	Within one week of a known clinical insult or new or worsening respiratory symptoms
Chest Imaging (Chest radiograph or CT)	Bilateral opacities not fully explained by effusions, lobar/lung collapse, or nodules
Origin of Edema	Respiratory failure not fully explained by cardiac failure or fluid overload

Table 12.2 ARDS Severity	
Mild	$200 \text{ mmHg} < PaO_2/F_IO_2 \leq 300 \text{ mmHg}$ with PEEP or CPAP $\geq 5 \text{ cmH}_2\text{O}$
Moderate	$100 \text{ mmHg} < PaO_2/F_IO_2 \leq 200 \text{ mmHg}$ with PEEP or CPAP $\geq 5 \text{ cmH}_2\text{O}$
Severe	$PaO_2/F_IO_2 \leq 100 \text{ mmHg}$ with PEEP or CPAP $\geq 5 \text{ cmH}_2\text{O}$

Precipitating Factors

Table 12.3 shows that some recognized triggers for ARDS cause direct lung injury, while others are extra-thoracic or systemic disorders.

Table 12.3 Common Risk Factors for ARDS	
Direct Lung Injury	**Indirect Lung Injury**
Pneumonia	Sepsis
Aspiration of gastric contents	Shock
Pulmonary contusion	Acute pancreatitis
Near drowning	Multiple trauma
Inhalation injury	Drug overdose
Fat embolism	Transfusion of blood products

Pathophysiology

ARDS is caused by acute lung injury that leads to abnormal pulmonary capillary permeability, alveolar flooding, and loss of surfactant. Studies using computed tomography (CT) imaging have identified three types of alveoli in patients with ARDS. Some are filled with edema fluid, others are collapsed (atelectatic), and some appear to be normal. In a supine patient, CT typically shows that the dependent, dorsal regions of the lungs are densely consolidated and airless, while the non-dependent, ventral areas are air-filled. Atelectatic alveoli populate the transition zone between these two regions.

Not surprisingly, during mechanical ventilation, most of the delivered gas goes to the open, relatively normal alveoli. The remainder enters previously atelectatic alveoli that are opened or "recruited" by the pressure applied during the mechanical breath. None of the delivered volume gets to the densely consolidated areas of the lungs. So, in effect, ARDS patients have very small lungs, and this is a key pathophysiological feature.

Respiratory Mechanics

Lung volume can increase only when sufficient pressure is supplied to overcome the elastic recoil of the respiratory system. Recall that elastic recoil or "stiffness" is inversely related to compliance (C), which is the change in lung volume (ΔV) divided by the required change in transmural pressure (ΔP_{TM}).

$$C = \Delta V / \Delta P_{TM} \qquad (12.1)$$

In patients with ARDS, lung and respiratory system compliance are reduced because extra pressure is needed to recruit atelectatic alveoli and because even modest volume changes over-distend the relatively small number of gas-filled alveoli.

Gas Exchange

One of the major defining features of ARDS is arterial hypoxemia that is resistant or refractory to high inspired oxygen concentrations. This is caused by the perfusion of fluid-filled and atelectatic alveoli, which produces a right-to-left intra-pulmonary shunt. As the proportion of the cardiac output passing through unventilated alveoli (the shunt fraction) rises, increases in F_1O_2 have less and less effect on PaO_2, and the P/F ratio falls.

The lack of ventilation to some alveoli means that other alveoli must receive too much. At the same time, the high pressure within these alveoli compresses the alveolar capillaries and reduces or stops blood flow. Over-ventilated and under- or non-perfused alveoli generate alveolar dead space, which increases the ratio of physiologic dead space to tidal volume (V_D/V_T). As V_D/V_T increases, alveolar volume and alveolar ventilation fall, and less CO_2 is excreted by the lungs. The relationship between V_D/V_T, minute ventilation ($\dot{V}_E$), and CO_2 excretion ($\dot{V}eCO_2$) can be expressed as:

$$\dot{V}eCO_2 \propto \dot{V}_E \times \left(1 - V_D/V_T\right) \qquad (12.2)$$

This shows that $\dot{V}_E$ must increase with V_D/V_T in order to maintain the same rate of CO_2 excretion and keep $PaCO_2$ constant. The high V_D/V_T explains why patients with ARDS have an abnormally elevated $\dot{V}_E$ requirement and why low tidal volume ventilation (see later in this chapter) is often accompanied by hypercapnia.

Mechanical Ventilation

Ventilatory support for the patient with ARDS has two major goals:

• Maintain adequate oxygenation
• Minimize ventilator-induced lung injury

Adequate Oxygenation

If you think about it, "adequate oxygenation" is a really vague term. What does it mean? In patients with ARDS, most physicians adjust F_1O_2 and PEEP, and, if necessary, use ancillary therapies to keep the arterial hemoglobin saturation (SaO_2) in the range of 91–93%. Given the sigmoid shape of the oxygen–hemoglobin dissociation curve, this goal is reasonable because it prevents small decrements in gas exchange from causing a precipitous fall in SaO_2. Although it's easy to continuously monitor SaO_2 using pulse oximetry (SpO_2), is this really the best measure of "oxygenation"?

Remember from Chapter 9 that hemoglobin saturation is only one factor that determines the oxygen content of arterial blood (CaO_2). If the very small volume of dissolved O_2 is neglected, CaO_2 (in ml of O_2 per dl of blood) is the product of the volume of O_2 carried by one gram (g) of fully saturated hemoglobin (1.34 ml/g), the hemoglobin concentration (Hb; g/dl), and the fractional hemoglobin saturation ($SaO_2/100$).

$$CaO_2 = 1.34 \times Hb \times SaO_2 \, / \, 100 \qquad (12.3)$$

But there's something even more important than O_2 content, and that's the rate at which O_2 is delivered to the tissues and organs of the body. Oxygen delivery ($\dot{D}O_2$) is expressed in terms of ml of O_2 per minute and is calculated by multiplying the arterial O_2 content by the cardiac output (CO).

$$\dot{D}O_2 = CaO_2 \times CO \qquad (12.4)$$

Substituting Equation 12.3 into Equation 12.4 gives us:

$$\dot{D}O_2 = \left(1.34 \times Hb \times SO_2 \, / \, 100 \times 10\right) \times CO \qquad (12.5)$$

Note that the components of O_2 content have been multiplied by a factor of 10 to convert ml/dl to ml/L. Now, when we multiply by CO (in L/min), $\dot{D}O_2$ will be in units of ml/min.

It's logical (although unproven) that ensuring adequate O_2 delivery is a more important and appropriate goal than simply maintaining the SaO_2 on the top portion of the dissociation curve. Focusing on O_2 delivery also helps us to remember that hemoglobin saturation is relatively unimportant. Since Equation 12.5 uses the *fractional* saturation ($SaO_2/100$), you can see that a small change in hemoglobin concentration or cardiac output affects O_2 delivery more than a larger change in SaO_2. For example, SaO_2 would have to increase from 80% to 90% to produce the same change in O_2 delivery as an increase in hemoglobin concentration from 8 to 9 g/dl or an increase in CO from 6.0 to 6.75 L/min. This is especially important because PEEP often reduces venous return, LV preload, and cardiac output. Increasing SaO_2 from 80% to 90% by raising PEEP from 10 to 15 cmH$_2$O might make *you* feel good, but it's unlikely to help your patient if it also causes a significant fall in cardiac output and systemic oxygen delivery.

The main obstacle to monitoring O_2 delivery, of course, is that it's not nearly as convenient as simply watching the continuous SpO_2 display. It requires the repeated measurement of hemoglobin concentration and cardiac output—and then there's that equation. Measuring hemoglobin concentration obviously isn't a problem, and cardiac output can now be assessed using a number of minimally invasive or noninvasive techniques. But here's the thing. You don't really need to calculate O_2 delivery. All you need to do is follow cardiac output or stroke volume as you increase PEEP. If there's a big drop, try to correct it with fluid boluses. As we'll discuss, PEEP does more than reduce shunt fraction and increase PaO_2 and SaO_2. It also plays an important role in limiting lung injury from mechanical ventilation, so some tradeoff between O_2 delivery and lung protection is often necessary.

A bigger problem is that we currently have no accurate way of determining whether O_2 delivery is "adequate." That's why I've intentionally used such an inexact term. Furthermore, since blood flow and metabolic rate vary considerably throughout the body, adequate O_2 delivery differs from one organ or tissue to another. Unfortunately, the best we can do is watch for signs of total body hypoxia, such as impaired organ function, elevation of the serum lactate concentration, and reduced central venous ($S\overline{cv}O_2$) or mixed venous ($S\overline{v}O_2$) hemoglobin saturation. When these signs are present, you should consider augmenting O_2 delivery by transfusing red cells, increasing cardiac output, or both.

Ventilator-Induced Lung Injury

In the latter part of the 20th century, studies in animals and humans provided convincing evidence that mechanical ventilation itself can cause lung injury and worsen or perpetuate ARDS. This so-called *ventilator-induced lung injury* (VILI) was shown to result from both alveolar over-distention during mechanical inflation and the repeated recruitment and de-recruitment of terminal respiratory units during each respiratory cycle. This led to the concept of "protective lung ventilation," in which tidal volume and PEEP are adjusted to avoid alveolar over-distention while maintaining the recruitment achieved during positive pressure breaths.

Tidal Volume

Low tidal volume ventilation has been the standard of care since 2000, when a prospective, randomized trial by the Acute Respiratory Distress Syndrome Network (ARDSnet) showed that patients receiving a tidal volume ≤6 ml/kg of ideal body weight (IBW) that maintained a plateau pressure ≤30 cmH$_2$O had significantly lower mortality than those receiving a tidal volume of 12 ml/kg IBW.

Any decrease in tidal volume must raise V_D/V_T, which further impairs CO_2 excretion and increases the minute ventilation needed to maintain a given PaCO$_2$ (Equation 12.2). That's why large drops in tidal volume should be avoided. Instead, there should be a stepwise reduction in tidal volume until the target of 6 ml/kg IBW is reached. At each step, arterial PCO$_2$ and pH are measured and respiratory rate (and minute ventilation) is increased as needed. Even with this stepwise approach, respiratory rate often cannot be increased sufficiently to maintain PaCO$_2$ within the normal range. Fortunately, this so-called permissive hypercapnia is usually well-tolerated. If necessary, intermittent boluses of IV sodium bicarbonate can be used to keep the arterial pH above 7.20.

Positive End-Expiratory Pressure

Since the initial description of ARDS in 1967, PEEP has been an essential part of management. By increasing end-expiratory lung volume, PEEP opens or "recruits" collapsed alveoli, thereby reducing shunt fraction and increasing PaO$_2$ and SaO$_2$. Although PEEP was mentioned in the previous section on "oxygenation," I will focus on it here because of its potential to improve lung compliance and reduce the cyclical opening and closing of alveoli that leads to lung injury.

Unfortunately, PEEP can also have two important detrimental effects. First, PEEP may reduce venous return, LV preload and stroke volume, and cardiac output (Chapter 3). This means that PEEP may improve PaO_2, SaO_2, and O_2 content while decreasing oxygen delivery to the tissues. Second, PEEP-induced elevation of end-expiratory pressure and volume may worsen lung injury by contributing to alveolar over-distention during a mechanical breath.

Three large, prospective trials that randomized ARDS patients to high or low PEEP were unable to show a difference in survival rates. This could mean that the level of PEEP really doesn't matter. Alternatively, it could mean that this "one size fits all" approach ignores the need to select PEEP based on the characteristics, extent, and duration of each patient's lung disease. Since the volume of "recruitable" lung has been shown to vary widely among patients, I think the second possibility is much more likely.

Unfortunately, there is no well-accepted method of identifying the level of PEEP that optimizes gas exchange while minimizing cyclical alveolar recruitment-de-recruitment and over-distention. This elusive ideal pressure is often referred to as "best PEEP." Attempts to individualize PEEP have focused primarily on techniques that assess respiratory mechanics, gas exchange, or both. The most commonly used methods are listed in Table 12.4. It's important to recognize that the impact of most of these techniques on any meaningful patient outcome has never been studied.

Before I describe each approach, I want to review two important concepts: recruitment maneuvers and PEEP titration. A *recruitment maneuver* is performed by applying high levels of positive pressure for a short period of time. For example, pressure-control breaths might be used to provide a PEEP of 30 cmH_2O for two minutes, while driving pressure is set to maintain the previously set tidal volume. The goal is to maximize alveolar recruitment, which can hopefully be maintained on a much lower PEEP setting. To this end, recruitment maneuvers are often followed by *decremental PEEP titration* (Figure 12.1).

Table 12.4 Methods of Selecting "Best PEEP"	
Gas exchange	PEEP is set at the lowest level needed to maintain adequate SpO_2.
	PEEP is selected to maximize SpO_2 or systemic O_2 delivery.
	PEEP is chosen to maximize CO_2 excretion or minimize alveolar or physiologic dead space.
Respiratory mechanics	PEEP is chosen to maximize respiratory system compliance.
	PEEP is set to maintain the "stress index" between 0.9 and 1.1.
	PEEP is set just above the lower inflection point of the pressure–volume curve.
Table	PEEP is chosen from a table listing combinations of F_iO_2 and PEEP.

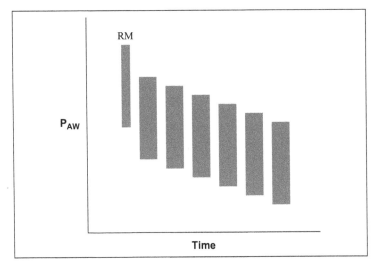

Figure 12.1 The airway pressure (P_{AW}) gradient of pressure control breaths during a recruitment maneuver (RM) and subsequent decremental PEEP titration. The top and bottom of each block represents end-inspiratory and end-expiratory pressure, respectively, at each PEEP level.

At each PEEP level, respiratory mechanics, gas exchange, or both, are assessed, and the results are used to select best PEEP. Alternatively, best PEEP can be based on measurements during stepwise increases in PEEP (incremental titration) without a recruitment maneuver. It's important to recognize, though, that both animal and human studies have shown that, at the same PEEP level, mechanics and gas exchange are much better following a recruitment maneuver.

Methods Assessing Gas Exchange

Least PEEP By far, the most common way of setting PEEP is to simply titrate it up or down based on the F_IO_2 and SpO_2. If F_IO_2 is high, PEEP is increased until a minimum SpO_2 (often 90–93%) is reached. As the patient improves, PEEP is reduced before, after, or with F_IO_2 in order to keep SpO_2 within this same range. This is often referred to as the "least PEEP" method, because the lowest possible PEEP is used to achieve a predetermined SpO_2.

There are several advantages to this approach. It's easy to do, PEEP is repeatedly assessed and adjusted throughout the course of the disease, and there is a reasonable correlation between SpO_2 and alveolar recruitment. On the other hand, PEEP is not directly linked with alveolar recruitment because the selected level is dependent on the F_IO_2. For example, best PEEP will be very different depending on whether a patient is receiving an F_IO_2 of 1.0 or 0.5. Furthermore, there is no mechanism for detecting alveolar recruitment-de-recruitment or over-distention.

Highest SpO_2 or $\dot{D}O_2$ A variant of the least PEEP approach is to perform incremental or decremental PEEP titration and identify the level that maximizes

SpO_2 or systemic oxygen delivery. As discussed previously, I believe that oxygen delivery is a much more appropriate target. Unfortunately, calculating oxygen delivery at multiple PEEP levels is time-consuming and requires repeated measurements of cardiac output. Titrating PEEP based on SpO_2 takes relatively little time, but like the least PEEP approach, best PEEP depends on F_iO_2, and there is no way to assess for PEEP-induced VILI.

Highest CO_2 Excretion and Lowest Dead Space Alternatively, ventilation can be assessed instead of oxygenation. Volume capnography continuously displays exhaled volume versus the expired CO_2 fractional concentration (FCO_2) or partial pressure (PCO_2) (Chapter 9). These data can be used to determine the volume of CO_2 exhaled per breath and per minute, the volume of the physiologic and alveolar dead space, and several dead-space-to-volume ratios. Alveolar recruitment augments CO_2 excretion by increasing the surface area of the gas–blood interface and reduces alveolar and physiologic dead space by diverting gas from previously over-ventilated alveoli. Alveolar over-distension, on the other hand, leads to excessive alveolar volume and reduced capillary blood flow, which generates high $\dot{V}/\dot{Q}$ regions, increases alveolar and physiologic dead space, and reduces CO_2 excretion. Accordingly, best PEEP is the level associated with the highest CO_2 excretion and the lowest alveolar and physiologic dead space (Figure 12.2).

Methods Assessing Respiratory Mechanics
All three techniques listed in Table 12.4 are based on the concept that alveolar recruitment increases lung compliance by distributing the tidal volume to

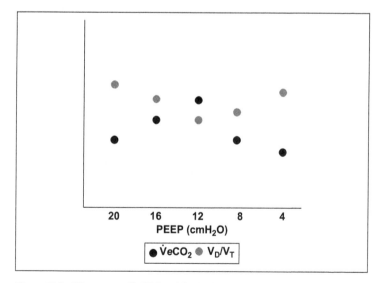

Figure 12.2 CO_2 excretion ($\dot{V}eCO_2$) and the dead space to tidal volume ratio (V_D/V_T) during decremental PEEP titration. In this example, best PEEP is 12 cmH_2O because it corresponds to the highest $\dot{V}e\ CO_2$ and the lowest V_D/V_T.

more alveoli, and that compliance falls as the lungs are stretched by alveolar over-distention.

Highest Compliance One method of determining best PEEP is to calculate respiratory system compliance from measurements of plateau and end-expiratory pressure (Chapter 9) during stepwise PEEP titration. The level that produces the highest compliance is best PEEP (Figure 12.3). Alternatively, dynamic compliance (C_{DYN}) can be used. "Dynamic compliance" is an oxymoron (think "jumbo shrimp") because compliance can only be measured under the static condition of zero gas flow. Nevertheless, this term has been around for decades and is unlikely to go away. It is calculated by dividing the delivered tidal volume (V_T) by the difference between the peak (P_{PEAK}) and the total end-expiratory pressure ($PEEP_T$) during a passive, volume-set breath.

$$C_{DYN} = V_T / \left(P_{PEAK} - PEEP_T \right) \tag{12.6}$$

The advantage of substituting dynamic for true "static" compliance is that it can be measured without performing an end-inspiratory pause, and many ventilators automatically calculate it on a breath-by-breath basis.

A large, randomized trial recently reported higher patient mortality when PEEP was adjusted to maximize compliance. Although several explanations have been proposed, this method of choosing PEEP cannot currently be recommended.

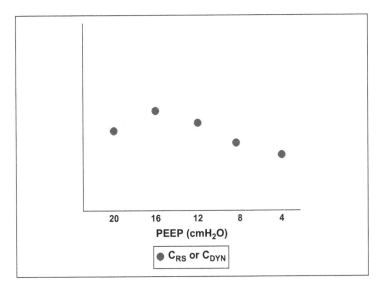

Figure 12.3 Respiratory system (static) compliance (C_{RS}) or dynamic compliance (C_{DYN}) during decremental PEEP titration. In this example, best PEEP is 16 cmH$_2$O because it corresponds to the highest compliance.

Optimal Stress Index During a mechanical breath, the pressure needed to balance the elastic recoil of the respiratory system increases with lung volume, and the slope of pressure versus volume equals the *elastance* (the reciprocal of compliance) of the respiratory system. If inspiratory flow is constant, time can be substituted for volume, and the pressure required to overcome viscous forces can be assumed to be constant. This means that the slope of airway pressure (P_{AW}) versus time during each mechanical breath approximates respiratory system elastance (Figure 12.4). If elastance is constant

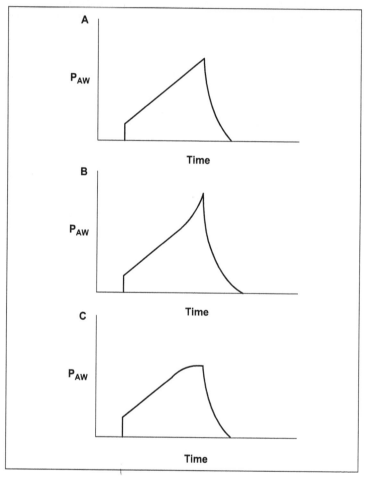

Figure 12.4 During a mechanical breath with constant inspiratory flow, the slope of the airway pressure (P_{AW})–time relationship equals the elastance of the respiratory system. If elastance remains constant (A), the slope is also constant. If the slope increases (B), elastance increases (compliance falls). If the slope decreases (C), elastance falls (compliance increases).

throughout inspiration, the slope of this relationship will also be constant (Figure 12.4A). If elastance increases (compliance falls), progressively more pressure is needed to balance elastic recoil, and the plot of P_{AW} vs. time will be convex (Figure 12.4B). If elastance falls (compliance increases), the curve will be concave (Figure 12.4C). Studies in both ARDS patients and animal models suggest that increasing elastance reflects alveolar over-distention (too much PEEP), whereas falling elastance reflects ongoing alveolar recruitment during inspiration and presumed de-recruitment during expiration (insufficient PEEP).

Although a significant change in elastance can sometimes be determined visually, the degree of convexity or concavity has also been quantified by fitting the P_{AW}–time curve to a power equation containing three variables (a, b, and c) and the inspiratory time (T_I):

$$P_{AW} = a \cdot T_I^b + c \qquad (12.7)$$

In this equation, the coefficient b is referred to as the "stress index" and reflects the slope of the P_{AW}–time curve. If b = 1, the curve is straight, indicating no change in elastance during the mechanical breath. If b > 1, elastance increases, and if b < 1, elastance falls during inspiration. At least one ventilator manufacturer has incorporated software to constantly calculate the stress index. Using this method, PEEP may be adjusted up or down to maintain the stress index between 0.9 and 1.1.

Lower Inflection Point In many ARDS patients, the plot of volume versus pressure, when measured in the absence of gas flow, has a characteristic S-shaped appearance (Figure 12.5). Since the slope of this curve equals compliance,

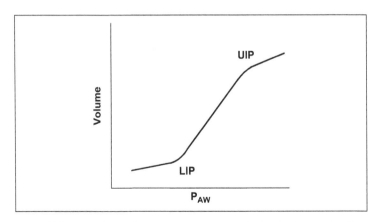

Figure 12.5 A plot of lung volume versus airway pressure (P_{AW}) in the absence of gas flow. The slope of the curve equals respiratory system compliance. The lower inflection point (LIP) may indicate the pressure needed for optimal alveolar recruitment (best PEEP). The upper inflection point (UIP) may identify optimal end-inspiratory pressure.

some investigators have equated the abrupt increase in slope at the "lower inflection point" (LIP) with the pressure needed to recruit all available alveoli (i.e., best PEEP). Using the same reasoning, flattening of the curve at the "upper inflection point" (UIP) indicates alveolar over-distention and suggests an excessively high tidal volume.

Since it's very difficult and time-consuming to plot a static volume–pressure curve in patients with ARDS, a "real-time" curve generated during a passive mechanical breath with slow, constant flow can be used instead. This "quasi-static" technique (another oxymoron) minimizes the pressure needed to overcome viscous forces and simulates a static volume–pressure curve.

This method of determining best PEEP has a number of major drawbacks that have limited its use. First, accurate determination of the LIP requires that measurements be performed on zero PEEP. This is potentially hazardous in patients with ARDS, especially if repeated measurements are performed. Second, even when performed correctly, there is no discernable LIP in a significant portion of patients. Finally, some studies suggest that alveolar recruitment continues well beyond the LIP.

The "Table" Method

I have included the "table" method approach to PEEP selection because many trainees mistakenly think that it's evidence-based. I'm talking about the tables pairing levels of F_IO_2 and PEEP that have been published with a number of randomized ARDS trials. Most are identical to the one used in the ARDSnet low tidal volume trial (Table 12.5). Since the investigators of these studies wanted to determine the effect of a specific intervention, it was essential that all other management be identical for both patient groups. This required a number of treatment protocols, including one linking F_IO_2 and PEEP. These tables were developed by the investigators to standardize care. They are not an evidence-based method for selecting the appropriate level of PEEP.

Putting It All Together

My recommendations for initial ventilator settings in patients with ARDS are shown in Table 12.6.

I use the CMV mode and volume-set breaths because this combination provides a guaranteed minute ventilation while allowing the patient to easily increase it if necessary. Both volume control (VC) and adaptive pressure control (aPC) breaths are acceptable. Pressure control (PC) breaths should be used with caution because tidal volume can vary with changes in compliance, resistance, and patient effort. If you choose VC breaths, increase inspiratory flow as needed to optimize patient comfort and ventilator synchrony

Table 12.5 Permitted F_IO_2–PEEP Combinations

F_IO_2	0.3	0.4	0.4	0.5	0.5	0.6	0.7	0.7	0.7	0.8	0.9	0.9	0.9	1.0	1.0	1.0	1.0
PEEP	5	5	8	8	10	10	10	12	14	14	14	16	18	18	20	22	24

Table 12.6 Initial Ventilator Settings for Patients with ARDS

Mode	CMV
Breath type	VC or aPC
Tidal volume	≤6 ml/kg IBW*
Respiratory rate	12
F_iO_2	1.0
PEEP	5.0 cmH$_2$O

*As needed to keep P_{PLAT} ≤ 30 cmH$_2$O

CMV = continuous mandatory ventilation; VC = volume control; aPC = adaptive pressure control; IBW = ideal body weight

(Chapter 11). If aPC is used, monitor the inspiratory pressure gradient to detect excessive patient work of breathing (Chapter 11, Figure 11.6).

Always start with an F_iO_2 of 1.0, because this maximizes your ability to quickly correct arterial hypoxemia. If possible, F_iO_2 can be reduced later based on PaO$_2$ and SpO$_2$.

PEEP can initially be set at 5 cmH$_2$O, but best PEEP should be determined as quickly as possible. Although none of the methods listed in Table 12.4 have been shown to improve patient morbidity or mortality, a few are more evidence-based than the others. In particular, several groups of investigators have quantified the extent of alveolar recruitment and over-distention in ARDS patients by performing CT after a recruitment maneuver and at each level during decremental PEEP titration. In these studies, the level of PEEP that maximized CO$_2$ excretion and minimized dead space correlated with optimal alveolar recruitment.

I recommend the following approach:

• If possible, measure baseline cardiac output.
• Perform a recruitment maneuver for 2–3 minutes using 30 cmH$_2$O PEEP and a pressure-control breath set to deliver a tidal volume ≤6 ml/kg IBW.
• Return to volume-set breaths with a PEEP of 24 cmH$_2$O. After 10 minutes, measure CO$_2$ excretion, V_D/V_T or both.
• Reduce PEEP in steps of 4 cmH$_2$O and repeat measurements after about 10 minutes at each level. The decremental PEEP titration is stopped when CO$_2$ excretion falls, when V_D/V_T increases, or when a PEEP level of 8 cmH$_2$O has been reached.
• Perform a second recruitment maneuver, then resume volume-set ventilation with PEEP set at the level corresponding to the highest CO$_2$ excretion and/or lowest V_D/V_T (best PEEP).
• Measure cardiac output. If there has been a significant fall, attempt to restore it to baseline with volume boluses.
• Reduce F_iO_2 until SpO$_2$ is in the 90–92% range.
• Repeat this process once a day.

Table 12.7 Ancillary Therapies for ARDS	
Ventilatory	**Non-Ventilatory**
High I:E ventilation	Prone positioning
• Conventional breaths	Neuromuscular blockade
• Bi-level ventilation	Inhaled vasodilators
• Airway pressure release ventilation	Extracorporeal membrane oxygenation

Ancillary Therapies

In most patients with ARDS, adequate oxygenation and lung protection can be maintained with low tidal volume ventilation using volume-set breaths, high F_IO_2, and best PEEP. Some patients, though, require ancillary therapies, and these can be divided into ventilatory and non-ventilatory types (Table 12.7). All of the listed therapies may increase PaO_2 and SaO_2, and experimental data suggest that several may improve patient survival.

Ventilatory Therapies

I will briefly review these techniques for the sake of completeness. However, since none have been shown in improve patient outcome and all have the potential to reduce systemic oxygen delivery and worsen ventilator-induced lung injury, I don't recommend them.

High I:E Ventilation

Recall that the ratio of inspiratory to expiratory time (I:E) is normally much less than one. That is, the duration of inspiration is usually a fraction of the time between breaths. As the I:E ratio increases, so does the mean alveolar pressure (MAP), which is the alveolar pressure averaged over the entire respiratory cycle. In general, an increase in MAP improves PaO_2 and SaO_2. An I:E ratio greater than 1.0 is referred to as *inverse ratio ventilation* (IRV).

Most often, the I:E ratio is increased by prolonging the set inspiratory time (Figure 12.6). Alternatively, on ventilators that require a set peak flow during VC breaths, an end-inspiratory pause can be added to produce the desired ratio.

Another option is to use bi-level ventilation, which is available on most ventilators. As discussed in Chapter 5, the bi-level mode alternates between a high (P_H) and a low (P_L) clinician-selected airway pressure, and patients may trigger spontaneous breaths at both levels (see Figure 5.3). The clinician also selects the duration of P_H and P_L, which determines the I:E ratio. Airway pressure release ventilation (APRV) is a variant of bi-level ventilation that uses a high P_H:P_L ratio.

By increasing MAP, high I:E ratios, like PEEP, increase pleural pressure, which can reduce venous return, cardiac output, and blood pressure. These effects become especially prominent when insufficient expiratory time causes

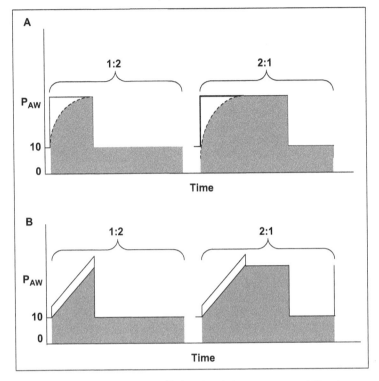

Figure 12.6 Plots of airway pressure (P_{AW}) vs. time during pressure control (A) and volume control (B) breaths with an I:E ratio of 1:2 and 2:1. The shaded areas equal mean alveolar pressure (MAP), which increases with I:E ratio and PEEP.

dynamic hyperinflation and intrinsic PEEP. That's why it's essential that cardiac output be monitored and both the beneficial and detrimental effects of high I:E ventilation be considered before abandoning more conventional forms of mechanical ventilation.

Non-Ventilatory Therapies

Prone Positioning

Physiology

It has long been recognized that turning patients with ARDS from the supine to the prone position usually increases PaO_2 and SaO_2. This was initially thought to result simply from the effect of gravity on lung perfusion. That is, the position change was assumed to reduce the shunt fraction by decreasing blood flow to the unventilated, fluid-filled or atelectatic alveoli in the dorsal, previously dependent regions and increasing flow to ventral, well-ventilated, and newly dependent alveoli. As usual, it turns out that things are a bit more complicated.

Studies in ARDS patients and in animal models of acute lung injury have revealed two key results of prone positioning. First, CT scans show that, within a short period of time, consolidation and atelectasis move from the dorsal to the now-dependent, ventral portions of the lungs. Second, in the prone position, most of the pulmonary blood flow is still directed to the non-dependent, dorsal lung regions. Taken together, this means that prone positioning improves arterial oxygenation by increasing the ventilation of persistently well-perfused dorsal lung regions.

Animal studies have also shown that prone positioning reduces the injurious effects of mechanical ventilation. Although there are several possible reasons for this, the most likely is that pleural pressure (P_{PL}) is much more uniform in the prone than in the supine position. Recall from Chapter 3 that lung transmural pressure ($P_{L_{TM}}$) is the difference between the pressure inside (alveolar pressure; P_{ALV}) and outside (pleural pressure; P_{PL}) the alveoli.

$$P_{L_{TM}} = P_{ALV} - P_{PL} \qquad (12.8)$$

In the supine position, P_{PL} is much greater (less negative or even positive) over the dorsal surfaces than over the ventral surfaces of the lungs. Because P_{ALV} is fairly uniform, $P_{L_{TM}}$ and alveolar volume progressively increase from the dorsal to the ventral portions of the lungs. This predisposes to alveolar collapse in dorsal lung regions and over-distention in ventral regions. During mechanical ventilation, cyclical opening and closing of collapsed lung units and inflation of already distended alveoli lead to lung injury.

In the prone position, there is little difference in P_{PL} and $P_{L_{TM}}$ between the non-dependent and dependent regions of the lungs, and this causes alveolar distending pressures and volumes to be much more uniform. This, in turn, is thought to reduce alveolar over-distention and cyclical recruitment and de-recruitment.

Clinical Evidence

Despite evidence that it reduces ventilator-induced lung injury, it has been difficult to prove that prone positioning, like low tidal volume ventilation, reduces mortality. Since 2001, there have been five large, prospective trials in which patients with ARDS have been randomized to supine or intermittent prone positioning (Table 12.8).

In the first four trials, prone positioning did not confer a survival benefit, although several meta-analyses suggested that the most severely ill patients were most likely to benefit. In the fifth (and probably final) trial, published in 2013, 466 patients with moderate or severe ARDS (defined as PaO_2/F_iO_2 < 150 with PEEP ≥ 5 cmH$_2$O and F_iO_2 ≥ 0.6) were randomized to prone-positioning for at least 16 hours per day or to be left in the supine position. Daily prone positioning was continued until day 28 or until there was significant,

Table 12.8 Randomized Trials Comparing Supine and Prone Positioning

Year	2001	2004	2006	2009	2013
Patients	304	802	142	344	474
Mean PaO_2/F_IO_2	127	152	105	113	100
Average duration of prone positioning	7 hours for 5 days	9 hours for 4 days	17 hours for 10 days	18 hours for 8 days	17 hours for 4 days
Follow-up	6 months	3 months	Hospital discharge	6 months	3 months
Mortality: prone vs. supine	62.5% vs. 58.6%	43.3% vs. 42.2%	50% vs. 60%	47% vs. 52.3%	23.6% vs. 41%

predefined improvement in gas exchange while in the supine position. Three-month mortality was 23.6% in the prone group and 41.0% in the supine group (P < 0.001). This dramatic effect, and the failure of previous trials to demonstrate it, was attributed primarily to greater severity of illness and the long periods of daily proning. It is worth noting, however, that these factors were very similar in the two negative studies that preceded it. Furthermore, the investigators found that the mortality benefit of prone positioning did not vary with ARDS severity. Finally, the generalizability of these results must be questioned, since only 1,434 out of 3,449 potential subjects with ARDS were screened for the study, and of these, only 474 were randomized.

Neuromuscular Blockade

Physiology

Pharmacological paralysis can significantly increase the PaO_2 and SaO_2 of patients with severe ARDS. Although several mechanisms have been proposed, the associated increase in the saturation of mixed venous blood ($S\bar{v}O_2$) is probably the most important. Let's examine this mechanism.

$S\bar{v}O_2$ is directly proportional to systemic O_2 delivery ($\dot{D}O_2$) and inversely related to total body O_2 consumption ($\dot{V}O_2$).

$$S\bar{v}O_2 \propto \dot{D}O_2/\dot{V}O_2 \qquad (12.9)$$

If more O_2 is delivered to the tissues but consumption doesn't change, there is more O_2 "left over," so the mixed venous blood contains more O_2, and $S\bar{v}O_2$ rises. If O_2 delivery doesn't change but less is used, the result is the same: mixed venous O_2 content and $S\bar{v}O_2$ increase. Neuromuscular blockade increases $S\bar{v}O_2$ by preventing respiratory and skeletal muscle contraction, thereby reducing O_2 consumption.

Now look at Figure 12.7. In the presence of a large shunt fraction, SaO_2 is the weighted average of the saturation of blood leaving ventilated alveoli and the saturation of mixed venous blood that passes unchanged through the lungs. Therefore, any increase in $S\bar{v}O_2$ must increase SaO_2 and arterial O_2 content.

Clinical Evidence

In a multi-center, prospective trial, 340 patients with moderate to severe ARDS ($PaO_2/F_iO_2 < 150$ on PEEP ≥ 5 cmH_2O) were randomized to receive continuous cisatracurium or placebo for 48 hours. Ninety-day mortality was 31.6% in the cisatracurium group and 40.7% in the control group (p = 0.08). When adjusted for PaO_2/F_iO_2, the baseline Simplified Acute Physiology Score (SAPS) II, and plateau pressure, patients receiving cisatracurium had a hazard ratio for death at 90 days of 0.68 (confidence interval [CI] 0.48–0.98) when compared with the placebo group. As noted by the study authors, the mechanisms responsible for these beneficial effects remain the subject of speculation.

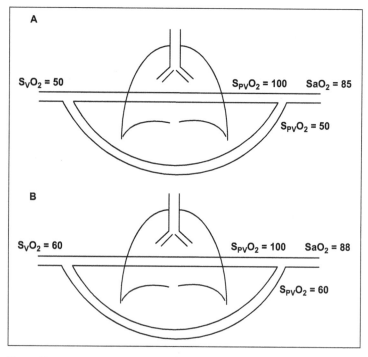

Figure 12.7 In patients with ARDS, SaO_2 is the weighted average of the saturation of pulmonary venous blood ($S_{PV}O_2$) passing through ventilated and unventilated lung regions (depicted as bypassing the lungs). Here, the shunt fraction is 30%, and SaO_2 increases from 85% to 88% when the mixed venous saturation (SvO_2) increases from 50% to 60%.

Inhaled Vasodilators

Physiology

Both nitric oxide and epoprostenol are potent vasodilators that can be administered through the ventilator circuit. Because they are given by inhalation, these drugs selectively dilate the pulmonary vessels in the ventilated regions of the lungs. This reduces local vascular resistance, which "steals" blood from unventilated regions, thereby reducing the shunt fraction and improving PaO_2 and SaO_2.

Clinical Evidence

Three moderate-sized randomized trials and several meta-analyses have shown that nitric oxide improves PaO_2 and SaO_2 in patients with ARDS but has no effect on mortality. Epoprostenol has been shown to be as effective as nitric oxide at improving arterial oxygenation at a fraction of the cost. No sufficiently powered trials have assessed the effect of epoprostenol on patient morbidity or mortality.

Extracorporeal Membrane Oxygenation (ECMO)

Physiology

Extracorporeal support for severe, refractory hypoxemia is performed using a veno-venous circuit (Figure 12.8). Blood is removed from the inferior

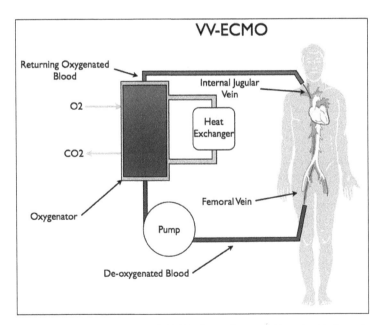

Figure 12.8 During veno-venous ECMO, blood is usually removed from the right femoral vein and returned through the right internal jugular vein. The ECMO circuit consists of cannulae and tubing, a blood pump, an oxygenator, and a heat exchanger.

vena cava using a large-bore catheter inserted via the femoral vein, pumped through a membrane that allows oxygen to be added and carbon dioxide to be removed, reheated to body temperature, and returned to the superior vena cava through an internal jugular vein catheter. If flow through the circuit approaches the cardiac output, mechanical ventilation isn't needed for gas exchange, and the ventilator can be set at a low respiratory rate, tidal volume, and F_IO_2. ECMO would appear to be perfectly suited for ARDS patients because it maintains adequate gas exchange while minimizing mechanical ventilation and ventilator-induced lung injury. The downside, of course, is that ECMO is invasive and associated with a number of major complications, including thrombosis and embolism, major bleeding, hemolysis, and infection.

Clinical Evidence

In the only relevant prospective trial, 180 patients with "severe but potentially reversible" ARDS were randomized to receive conventional therapy or to be transferred to a single ECMO center. Six-month survival without severe disability was significantly greater in the patients transferred to the ECMO center (63% vs. 47%). Unfortunately, this trial was far from conclusive, because only 75% of the transferred patients actually received ECMO and because there were significant treatment differences between the two groups. Pending the results of truly randomized trials, veno-venous-ECMO should be considered only in patients dying from tissue and organ hypoxia.

Additional Reading

Bein T, Grasso S, Moerer O, et al. The standard of care of patients with ARDS: Ventilatory settings and rescue therapies for refractory hypoxemia. *Intensive Care Med*. 2016;42:699–711.

Fan E, Del Sorbo L, Goligher EC, et al. An official American Thoracic Society/European Society of Intensive Care Medicine/Society of Critical Care Medicine clinical practice guideline: Mechanical ventilation in adult patients with acute respiratory distress syndrome. *Am J Respir Crit Care Med*. 2017;195:1253–1263.

Hess DR. Recruitment maneuvers and PEEP titration. *Respir Care*. 2015;60:1688–1704.

Kallet RH. Should PEEP titration be based on chest mechanics in patients with ARDS? *Respir Care*. 2016;61:876–890.

MacSweeney R, McAuley DF. Acute respiratory distress syndrome. *Lancet*. 2016;338: 2416–2430.

Marini JJ, Josephs SA, Mechlin M, Hurford WE. Should early prone positioning be a standard of care in ARDS with refractory hypoxemia? *Respir Care*. 2016;61:818–829.

Munshi L, Rubenfeld G, Wunsch H. Adjuvants to mechanical ventilation for acute respiratory distress syndrome. *Intensive Care Med*. 2016;42:775–778.

Rittayamai N, Brochard L. Recent advances in mechanical ventilation in patients with acute respiratory distress syndrome. *Eur Respir Rev*. 2015;24:132–140.

Vieillard-Baron A, Matthay M, Teboul JL, et al. Experts' opinion on management of hemodynamics in ARDS patients: Focus on the effects of mechanical ventilation. *Intensive Care Med*. 2016;42:739–749.

Chapter 13

Severe Obstructive Lung Disease

Although COPD, asthma, bronchiectasis, and bronchiolitis have very different causes, clinical features, and therapies, they share the same underlying pathophysiology. They are referred to as *obstructive lung diseases* because airway narrowing causes increased resistance and slowing of expiratory gas flow. Mechanical ventilation of patients with severe obstructive lung disease often produces two problems that must be recognized and effectively managed: over-ventilation and dynamic hyperinflation.

Over-Ventilation

Here, I'm referring to excessive minute ventilation in patients with chronic, compensated hypercapnia that reduces the $PaCO_2$ below the *patient's baseline* (but not necessarily below normal). This causes alkalemia due to an apparent metabolic alkalosis. Over a period of several days, reduced renal bicarbonate reclamation and regeneration will decrease the serum bicarbonate concentration and return the blood pH toward normal. The problem is that this eliminates the metabolic compensation required for the patient to maintain their usual $PaCO_2$.

Let's look at an example. A patient with severe COPD has a baseline $PaCO_2$ of 80 mmHg, a serum bicarbonate concentration of 40 meq/L, and an arterial pH of 7.30. He is admitted to the ICU with a COPD exacerbation that has caused his $PaCO_2$ to increase to 100 mmHg and his pH to fall to 7.14. He is intubated and ventilated using CMV-VC with a set, mandatory rate of 18, and he does not trigger any spontaneous breaths. About a half-hour after intubation, blood gas measurements show a $PaCO_2$ of 60 mmHg, a calculated bicarbonate concentration of 40 meq/L, and a pH of 7.46. Several days later, his $PaCO_2$ is still 60 mmHg, but the bicarbonate concentration has fallen to 32 meq/L, and the pH has dropped to 7.38.

So what's the problem? The problem is that when you decide that the patient's respiratory status has returned to baseline and perform a spontaneous breathing trial, his $PaCO_2$ will acutely increase back to its baseline level of 80 mmHg, his pH will fall to 7.22, and he will be placed back on CMV. You can see that the patient will never get off the ventilator because he no longer has the metabolic compensation needed for his baseline minute ventilation and $PaCO_2$.

Fortunately, the vast majority of patients with chronic hypercapnia will maintain their baseline $PaCO_2$ during mechanical ventilation, *if you let them*. Unfortunately, as in the case I just described, an inappropriately high set respiratory rate and failure to recognize its consequences are common. Consequently, this is also a common cause of chronic ventilator-dependence in patients with severe obstructive lung disease.

So how do you avoid this problem? First, determine your patient's baseline $PaCO_2$. Look at their blood gas measurements for the past few years. If there aren't any, look at their serum bicarbonate (or total CO_2) concentrations. If they're chronically elevated, you can be pretty sure that the patient has chronic hypercapnia. You can estimate the baseline $PaCO_2$ by assuming that chronic respiratory acidosis causes the serum bicarbonate concentration to increase by about 4 meq/L (from 24 meq/L) for every 10 mmHg elevation (from 40 mmHg) in the $PaCO_2$. For example, a patient with a chronic serum bicarbonate concentration of 36 meq/L would be expected to have a $PaCO_2$ of about 70 mmHg. Second, make sure that you set a low mandatory rate. Many patients with chronic hypercapnia only need 6–10 breaths per minute. The best way to avoid over-ventilation is to make sure that the patient always triggers spontaneous breaths. This can easily be confirmed by noting that the total respiratory rate exceeds the set rate on the ventilator–user interface.

Dynamic Hyperinflation

Since a lot of time is needed for complete exhalation, patients with severe air flow obstruction are likely to receive or trigger another mechanical breath before the respiratory system has returned to its resting or equilibrium volume. This is referred to as *dynamic hyperinflation*, and this topic was covered in Chapter 10. The more end-expiratory lung volume exceeds the equilibrium volume, the greater the remaining elastic recoil and the higher the alveolar (elastic recoil) pressure. This end-expiratory alveolar pressure is called *total PEEP* ($PEEP_T$), and the difference between total and set (extrinsic) PEEP ($PEEP_E$) is called *intrinsic PEEP* ($PEEP_I$).

Both the presence and severity of air flow obstruction and dynamic hyperinflation can be determined by examining the flow–time curve on the ventilator user interface. As shown in Figure 13.1, as obstruction worsens, it takes more and more time for complete exhalation to occur. Dynamic hyperinflation and $PEEP_I$ must be present if a mechanical breath occurs before expiratory flow reaches zero.

As discussed in Chapter 3, both $PEEP_I$ and $PEEP_E$ increase pleural pressure (P_{PL}) and intramural right atrial pressure (PRA_{IM}) throughout the respiratory cycle. This reduces venous return, which can decrease cardiac output and blood pressure. It's long been recognized that hypotension is much more likely to occur with intrinsic than extrinsic PEEP, but it's important to understand that the type of PEEP is irrelevant. What matters is the clinical setting in

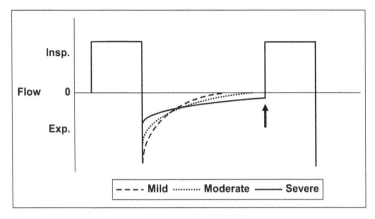

Figure 13.1 Inspiratory (Insp) and expiratory (Exp) flow curves in patients with mild, moderate, and severe obstructive lung disease. Dynamic hyperinflation and $PEEP_I$ are present when the next mechanical breath occurs before expiratory flow reaches zero (*arrow*).

which it occurs (Figure 13.2). Extrinsic PEEP is used to improve oxygenation in patients with ARDS. Since compliance is low, the increase in lung volume and P_{PL} produced by a given PEEP level is small, P_{PL} remains negative (subatmospheric) throughout inspiration, and hemodynamic effects are typically small or absent. On the other hand, since $PEEP_I$ occurs in patients with normal or high (emphysema) lung compliance, the same level of PEEP causes a larger increase in lung volume and P_{PL}, and adverse hemodynamic effects are common.

As dynamic hyperinflation worsens and $PEEP_I$ increases, patients with obstructive lung disease are more and more likely to develop hypotension. Although this may happen at any time, it's most common immediately after intubation, and there are several reasons for this. First, patients are often volume-depleted because empiric diuresis is commonly used in an attempt to treat possible congestive heart failure and stave off intubation. Second, sedative-hypnotics, narcotics, and anesthetics directly dilate systemic arterioles while eliminating respiratory distress–induced adrenergic activation. Finally, over-zealous manual bag-mask ventilation or an excessively high set respiratory rate may cause or worsen dynamic hyperinflation. By generating high levels of $PEEP_I$ and P_{PL}, this may markedly reduce venous return and even cause pulseless electrical activity (PEA).

Dynamic hyperinflation may also interfere with effective ventilator triggering by producing a "threshold load" on the respiratory muscles (Chapters 10 and 11). When the respiratory system is above its equilibrium volume, a patient trying to trigger a mechanical breath must first stop expiratory flow by generating pressure equal to $PEEP_I$. Additional pressure must then be supplied

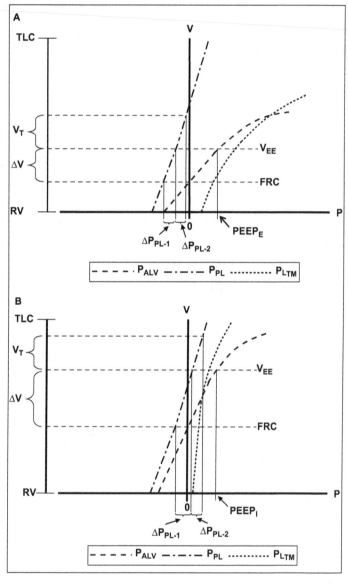

Figure 13.2 The relationship between lung volume and alveolar (P_{ALV}), pleural (P_{PL}), and lung transmural ($P_{L_{TM}}$) pressure in a patient with low lung compliance and extrinsic PEEP ($PEEP_E$) (A), and a patient with obstructive lung disease, normal lung compliance, and intrinsic PEEP ($PEEP_I$) (B). PEEP causes a larger increase (ΔV) in end-expiratory volume (V_{EE}) and pleural pressure (ΔP_{PL-1}) when lung compliance is normal. During tidal inflation (V_T), P_{PL} is much more likely to be positive (ΔP_{PL-2}) when lung compliance is normal.

to lower airway pressure or the base flow sufficiently to trigger a mechanical breath.

Mechanical Ventilation

Recommended initial settings are shown in Table 13.1. As in other critically ill patients with respiratory failure, it's important to provide a guaranteed tidal volume and minute ventilation, so I recommend using the CMV mode with volume control (VC) or adaptive pressure control (aPC) breaths. It's also essential to correct arterial hypoxemia. Most patients have a modest supplemental oxygen requirement (e.g., 2–6 L/min) prior to intubation, and I routinely start these patients on an F_1O_2 of 0.5. If the patient has a higher oxygen requirement, an initial F_1O_2 of 1.0 is appropriate.

As previously discussed, it's important to start with a low mandatory rate that allows the patient to set their own minute ventilation. An unnecessarily high rate not only causes relative hypocapnia and bicarbonate excretion, it also reduces expiratory time and may precipitate or worsen dynamic hyperinflation and its hemodynamic consequences. Given the likelihood of dynamic hyperinflation, I do not use $PEEP_E$ in patients with severe obstructive lung disease.

Once mechanical ventilation has begun, assess for dynamic hyperinflation using the expiratory flow–time curve, measure $PEEP_1$ if dynamic hyperinflation is present, follow blood pressure closely, and obtain arterial blood gas measurements.

Reduce F_1O_2 as much as possible to maintain SpO_2 in the range of 91–93%. Even if dynamic hyperinflation is present, no changes in the initial set rate or tidal volume are needed as long as ventilation is sufficient to keep the arterial pH above 7.20 and blood pressure remains normal. Reduce the set rate if pH exceeds 7.35. If blood pressure is normal and the arterial pH is less than 7.20, increase the set rate as needed to maintain pH ≥ 7.20.

If the patient develops hypotension following intubation, it's important to consider other possible causes, even if dynamic hyperinflation is present. In general, the higher the $PEEP_1$, the more likely it is to be causing or contributing

Table 13.1 Initial Ventilator Settings for Patients with Severe Obstructive Lung Disease	
Mode	CMV
Breath type	VC or aPC
Tidal volume	6–8 ml/kg IBW
Respiratory rate	8
F_1O_2	0.5 or 1.0
PEEP	0 cmH$_2$O

CMV = continuous mandatory ventilation; VC = volume control; aPC = adaptive pressure control; IBW = ideal body weight

to the hypotension. Dynamic hyperinflation is unlikely to be a contributing factor if $PEEP_i$ is ≤5 cmH_2O. Intrinsic PEEP-induced hypotension can be diagnosed with certainty only if blood pressure rises rapidly during a brief period of spontaneous breathing. If clinically feasible and the patient has an arterial catheter, this can usually be determined by disconnecting the patient from the ventilator circuit for 10–15 seconds.

As discussed in Chapter 10, the treatment of intrinsic PEEP-induced hypotension must focus on two goals. First, extra-thoracic venous pressure must be increased by intravenous volume loading. This increases the gradient for venous return, which improves RV and LV preload and stroke volume. Second, dynamic hyperinflation must be reduced. Recall that this can be done by increasing expiratory flow (e.g., treating bronchospasm, clearing large-airway secretions, inserting a new, larger-diameter endotracheal tube) and by lengthening the time available for expiration by reducing the total respiratory rate, tidal volume, or both. Sometimes cardiac output and blood pressure can be restored only by sedating and pharmacologically paralyzing the patient and allowing the $PaCO_2$ to rise. If necessary, boluses of IV sodium bicarbonate can be given to keep the arterial pH ≥ 7.20.

Chapter 14

Right Ventricular Failure

Right ventricular (RV) failure is common in the ICU. *Chronic* RV failure is most often due to long-standing pulmonary hypertension. *Acute* RV failure can result from massive pulmonary embolism, ARDS, RV infarction, and acute LV failure. Finally, *acute-on-chronic* RV failure can be precipitated by any disorder that leads to an abrupt rise in pulmonary vascular resistance (PVR) and RV afterload. Common causes include pneumonia, exacerbation of chronic lung disease, and pulmonary embolism. As discussed in Chapter 3, mechanical ventilation and PEEP also increase RV afterload, so it's not surprising that they can trigger acute or acute-on-chronic RV failure. This chapter reviews the pathophysiology of RV failure, highlights the effects of mechanical ventilation and PEEP on the pulmonary circulation and RV, and provides physiology-based mechanical ventilation guidelines for patients with, or at risk for, RV failure.

Pathophysiology of RV Failure

In the absence of acute RV infarction, acute or acute-on-chronic RV failure (which I will refer to collectively as "acute RV failure") is most commonly precipitated by an abrupt increase in afterload. That's because neither the normal right ventricle, nor one that is hypertrophied due to chronic pulmonary hypertension, is capable of generating sufficient additional pressure to overcome even a relatively small increase in PVR.

Acute RV failure causes ventricular dilation and a rise in RV end-diastolic pressure and volume. This triggers a sequence of events that leads to further impairment of RV function and may progress to cardiogenic shock (Figure 14.1). Since both ventricles share a common wall (the septum), and their combined volume is limited by the pericardium, RV dilation causes the septum to flatten and shift toward the LV (Figure 14.2). This reduces LV size and compliance, which impairs diastolic filling. RV dilation may also cause or worsen tricuspid regurgitation. The combination of reduced RV systolic function and tricuspid regurgitation decreases RV stroke volume. This, in combination with impaired LV diastolic filling, decreases LV stroke volume, which, if sufficiently severe, leads to hypotension. At the same time, increased pressure-generation by the RV augments wall stress and oxygen demand while reducing coronary blood flow. This leads to RV ischemia, which reduces contractility and worsens RV dilation, RV systolic and LV diastolic function, and LV stroke volume. Systemic hypotension worsens this vicious cycle by further reducing coronary blood flow.

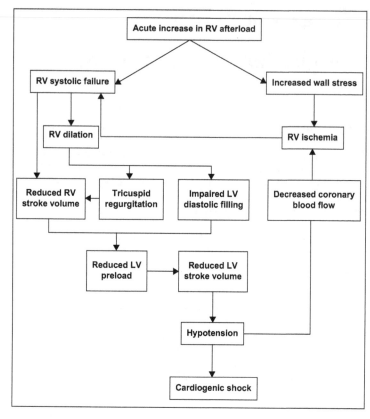

Figure 14.1 An acute rise in RV afterload may precipitate a series of events that ultimately leads to cardiogenic shock.

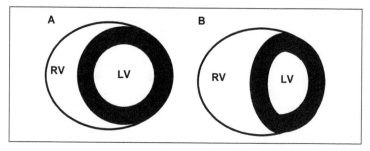

Figure 14.2 Representation of a short-axis, parasternal view from a transthoracic echocardiogram in a patient with (A) normal right ventricle (RV) and left ventricle (LV) and (B) severe RV dilation. RV pressure and volume overload causes the interventricular septum to shift toward the left ventricle.

Mechanical Ventilation and the RV

The effects of mechanical ventilation and PEEP on PVR and RV afterload were reviewed in Chapter 3. Here, I will only summarize the important points.

- RV afterload is proportional to PVR.
- PVR is proportional to lung transmural pressure (P_{LTM}), which is alveolar pressure (P_{ALV}) minus pleural pressure (P_{PL}).
- By increasing P_{LTM}, mechanical ventilation causes a cyclical increase in PVR and RV afterload.
- Extrinsic and intrinsic PEEP cause continuous elevation of end-expiratory and end-inspiratory P_{LTM}, which further increases PVR and RV afterload.
- The hemodynamic significance of these changes depends on the extent to which tidal ventilation and PEEP increase P_{LTM}, and on baseline ventricular function.
  - The change in P_{LTM} varies directly with the delivered tidal volume and the level of total PEEP, and inversely with lung compliance (Figure 14.3). In other words, a mechanical breath and PEEP will have a greater effect on RV afterload in a patient with low lung compliance (e.g., from pulmonary fibrosis).
  - The hemodynamic effect of a given rise in P_{LTM} will be greater in patients with impaired RV contractility or elevated RV afterload.

Guidelines for Mechanical Ventilation

Because of its adverse effects on RV afterload, mechanical ventilation should be avoided in patients with acute or chronic RV failure. If mechanical ventilation is absolutely necessary, the following recommendations are based on reducing the physiological effects listed previously.

- Non-invasive ventilation (Chapter 16) may be preferable to intubation because of the decreased need for sedating drugs, which may cause or worsen hypotension.
- Use low tidal volume ventilation; 6 ml/kg of ideal body weight is an appropriate target.
- Maintain a low plateau pressure (P_{PLAT}). Remember that P_{PLAT} is alveolar pressure at end-inspiration, so it's directly related to lung transmural pressure ($P_{ALV} - P_{PL}$) and PVR. Studies in ARDS patients suggest that the risk of acute RV failure is minimized when P_{PLAT} is maintained ≤27 mmHg.
- Since P_{LTM} (and PVR) falls as compliance increases, PEEP should be titrated to maximize alveolar recruitment in patients with ARDS (Chapter 12).
- PEEP should be set at zero in patients without ARDS.
- Assess for and minimize intrinsic PEEP (Chapter 10).
- Correct hypoxemia, hypercapnia, and acidemia. All three conditions cause pulmonary vasoconstriction, which increases PVR and RV afterload.

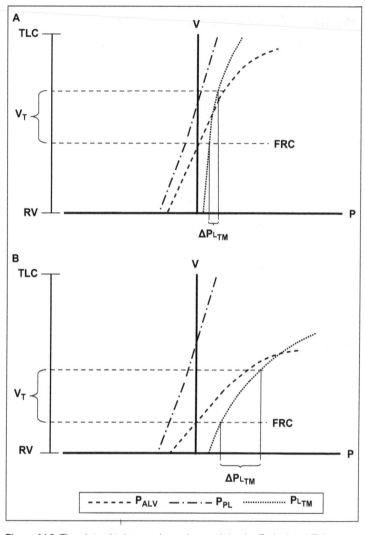

Figure 14.3 The relationship between lung volume and alveolar (P_{ALV}), pleural (P_{PL}), and lung transmural (PL_{TM}) pressure in a patient with normal (A) and decreased (B) lung compliance. The increase in lung transmural pressure (ΔPL_{TM}), pulmonary vascular resistance, and RV afterload varies directly with tidal volume (V_T) and PEEP and inversely with lung compliance.

Of course, it may be difficult to simultaneously achieve all of these goals. In particular, maintaining low tidal volume ventilation at a low P_{PLAT} is likely to precipitate or worsen arterial hypoxemia, hypercapnia, and acidemia. These abnormalities can often be at least partially corrected by increasing the F_IO_2, the set respiratory rate, or both.

Other Therapies

The following therapies are logical and often recommended, although no studies have been performed to evaluate their efficacy.

Optimize RV Preload

With the possible exception of patients with RV infarction, acute or acute-on-chronic RV failure is almost always accompanied by elevated RV preload. The magnitude of pressure and volume overload can be assessed by point-of-care cardiac ultrasound and by measuring central venous pressure (CVP). When confirmed, excessive RV preload should be treated with diuresis in an effort to reduce LV compression and improve LV diastolic filling. Serial ultrasound imaging and CVP measurements are essential to avoid over-diuresis and a significant drop in RV stroke volume. In many cases, right heart catheterization provides additional information that helps optimize RV preload, LV stroke volume, and cardiac output.

Vasopressors and Inotropes

Systemic blood pressure must be maintained to provide adequate blood flow to the heart and other vital organs. Norepinephrine is most often used in patients with acute RV failure because it increases cardiac contractility and systemic vascular resistance (SVR), with relatively little increase in heart rate or PVR.

If blood pressure is adequate, inotropes such as dobutamine or milrinone may improve hemodynamics by increasing RV contractility. The downside of both drugs is that they cause systemic vasodilation, which often leads to hypotension.

Pulmonary Vasodilators

Nebulized nitric oxide (NO) and epoprostenol are potent vasodilators that can rapidly and significantly reduce PVR in patients with RV failure. Because they are administered by inhalation and have a very short half-life, these drugs do not cause systemic vasodilation and hypotension.

Additional Reading

Harjolal VP, Mebazaa A, Celutkiene J, et al. Contemporary management of acute right ventricular failure: A statement from the Heart Failure Association and the Working Group on Pulmonary Circulation and Right Ventricular Function of the European Society of Cardiology. *Eur J Heart Fail*. 2016;18:226–241.

Krishnan S, Schmidt GA. Acute right ventricular dysfunction. *Chest*. 2015;147:835–846.

Chapter 15

Discontinuing Mechanical Ventilation

So far, you've read a great deal about when to start and how to manage mechanical ventilation. Now we're going to discuss when and how to remove or "wean" patients from the ventilator. While this may not seem as challenging (or exciting) as endotracheal intubation and selecting ventilator settings, the process of discontinuing mechanical ventilation is just as important. That's because unnecessary delays increase the incidence of hospital-acquired infections, lengthen ICU stay, and increase health care costs. On the other hand, stopping mechanical ventilation too soon exposes the patient to the risks associated with recurrent respiratory failure and re-intubation.

This chapter provides you with step-by-step instructions on how to discontinue mechanical ventilation. Although my goal is to help you avoid both delayed and premature extubation, as you'll see, this process is often more of an art than a science, and no one gets it right every time. I'll also provide an approach to the difficult-to-wean patient that emphasizes the identification and treatment of the underlying cause(s) of ventilator-dependence.

The Weaning Process

As shown in Figure 15.1, the process of discontinuing mechanical ventilation consists of four steps.

Step 1: Sedation Interruption

Sedation and analgesia are an essential and beneficial part of ICU care, but their benefits must be balanced by the fact that an impaired level of alertness delays weaning from mechanical ventilation. Studies have shown that routine, daily sedation-interruption allows the early identification of patients who are ready to resume spontaneous breathing and significantly decreases both the duration of mechanical ventilation and ICU length of stay.

Step 2: Determine Whether the Patient Is Ready to Begin the Weaning Process

This step requires that you understand why your patient required intubation and mechanical ventilation in the first place. As discussed in Chapter 7 and listed in Table 15.1, the reasons can be grouped into four major categories.

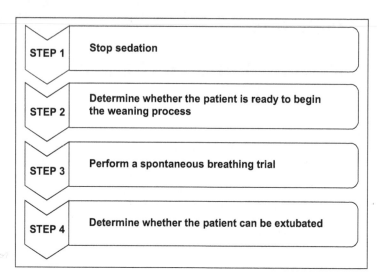

Figure 15.1 The four steps of the weaning process.

Table 15.1 Indications for Intubation and Mechanical Ventilation

Category	Causes	Examples
Acute or acute-on-chronic hypercapnia	Reduced respiratory drive	Toxic/metabolic encephalopathy
	Impaired transmission to the respiratory muscles	ALS, Guillain-Barre syndrome, myasthenia gravis, phrenic nerve injury
	Respiratory muscle weakness	Metabolic myopathy, polymyositis
	Severe lung or chest wall disease	COPD, asthma, pulmonary edema, morbid obesity
Refractory hypoxemia	Alveolar filling diseases	ARDS, pulmonary edema, pneumonia
Inability to protect the lower airway	Depressed level of consciousness plus vomiting risk	Toxic/metabolic encephalopathy plus upper GI bleeding or small-bowel obstruction
Upper airway obstruction	Anaphylaxis, epiglottitis, laryngeal mass, vocal cord paralysis	

ALS = amyotrophic lateral sclerosis; COPD = chronic obstructive pulmonary disease; ARDS = acute respiratory distress syndrome; GI = gastrointestinal

- Acute or acute-on-chronic hypercapnia
- Refractory hypoxemia
- Inability to protect the lower airway
- Upper airway obstruction

Every day, you need to assess how much improvement there has been in the disorder that led to intubation. If your therapy has been largely unsuccessful, there's no reason to think that your patient can be extubated. If, on the other hand, the original problem has resolved, or has at least significantly improved, your patient is probably ready to start the weaning process. While sedation is on hold, check to see whether your patient meets the general criteria shown in Box 15.1. If so, it's time to move on to the next step.

Step 3: Perform a Spontaneous Breathing Trial

Now it's time to see whether your patient can breathe on their own by performing a *spontaneous breathing trial* (SBT). This can be done using either a "T-piece" or low-level pressure support (PS) breaths, and these two methods are compared in Table 15.2. During a T-piece trial, the patient is removed from the ventilator, and the endotracheal tube is connected at a right angle to large-bore tubing (hence the name "T-piece") that carries high-flow, humidified gas. During a pressure support trial, the patient remains connected to the ventilator but only receives a small amount of inspiratory assistance (usually 5 cmH$_2$O), which helps to overcome the extra viscous forces created by the endotracheal tube and ventilator circuit.

As you can see from Table 15.2, there are lots of advantages to using PS trials. Most importantly, since the patient remains connected to the ventilator, you can easily monitor respiratory rate and tidal volume, and an alarm will sound when preset limits are reached. This gives PS trials a huge safety advantage. Pressure support trials also allow the patient to be suctioned more easily and eliminate the need (and the time required) for a respiratory therapist to repeatedly disconnect and reconnect the ventilator.

Box 15.1 Criteria for Beginning the Weaning Process

- Awake and alert when off sedation
- Adequate gas exchange
  - F$_I$O$_2$ ≤ 0.50
  - PEEP ≤ 8 cmH$_2$O
- Adequate ventilation
  - pH > 7.30
- Adequate hemodynamic status
  - No cardiac ischemia
  - No uncontrolled arrhythmias
  - No or stable, low-dose vasopressor requirement

F$_I$O$_2$ = fractional inspired oxygen concentration; PEEP = positive end-expiratory pressure

Table 15.2 Comparison of T-piece and Pressure Support Spontaneous Breathing trials

	T-piece	Pressure Support
Connected to ventilator	No	Yes
Inspiratory pleural pressure during breathing trial	Decreases	Increases
Provides supplemental oxygen	Yes	Yes
Compensates for extra viscous forces	No	Yes
Can add PEEP	No	Yes
Able to measure tidal volumes	No	Yes
Ventilator alarms active	No	Yes

PEEP = positive end-expiratory pressure

In fact, I use T-piece trials only when patients have severe left ventricular (LV) dysfunction. As discussed in Chapter 3, the increase in pleural pressure produced by a switch from spontaneous to mechanical ventilation actually assists the failing heart by reducing both LV preload and afterload. Patients with systolic heart failure may do well on a PS trial but then develop acute pulmonary edema after extubation. A T-piece trial subjects the heart to the same pleural pressures and the same preload and afterload that will be present after extubation. In this way, occult myocardial ischemia or decompensated LV failure usually declares itself prior to removal of the endotracheal tube.

Step 4: Determine If the Patient Is Ready for Extubation

Although there's no foolproof method of accurately predicting whether extubation will be successful, making sure that your patient meets all of the following criteria during a SBT will allow you to be right almost all of the time:

• The patient is awake, alert, and cooperative.
• The patient's spontaneous respiratory rate is ≤25 breaths per minute.
• The patient's spontaneous tidal volume is ≥300 ml.
• When asked, the patient is able to significantly increase his/her spontaneous tidal volume.

Blood gas measurements are not routinely needed prior to extubation. I do, however, measure pH and $PaCO_2$ when patients have chronic hypercapnia. I've learned the hard way that patients with a rising $PaCO_2$ can look very comfortable during an SBT.

There are two important questions that have not been addressed. The first is: How long should an SBT last? With great confidence, I can answer: "It depends." For example, a patient who is alert after being intubated for a drug overdose usually needs an SBT of no more than 5–10 minutes. The same is true for a healthy postoperative patient who has fully awakened from general anesthesia. On the other hand, most critical care physicians prefer a longer observation period (usually ½–1 hour) when patients have chronic lung or cardiac disease, neuromuscular disease, morbid obesity, or other disorders that predispose them to recurrent respiratory failure. Continuing a trial beyond one hour does not provide additional prognostic information. The second question is much easier to answer: What do you do when a patient does poorly on an SBT? Simply return them to their previous ventilator settings and try again in 12–24 hours.

Other Considerations

Once a patient has "passed" an SBT, you need to consider a few more issues before proceeding with extubation:

- Is the patient at risk for post-extubation laryngeal edema?
- Will the patient be able to effectively clear secretions from the airways following extubation?
- Does the patient have a "difficult airway" should the need for re-intubation arise?

Laryngeal Edema

The likelihood of post-extubation laryngeal edema and upper-airway obstruction increases with the duration of intubation. Prior airway trauma and multiple intubations are other important risk factors. Because laryngeal edema is very difficult to detect while the endotracheal tube is in place, a "cuff leak test" is often performed in patients who are at risk for this complication. This is done by deflating the endotracheal tube cuff and listening for the sound of an air leak during a mechanical breath. The theory is that significant laryngeal edema will prevent air from escaping even when the trachea is no longer sealed. Although this makes a lot of sense, the absence of an air leak is, unfortunately, fairly nonspecific. That is, many (most) patients without an air leak will have no sign of upper airway obstruction after extubation. Nevertheless, in high-risk patients, the absence of an air leak tells you that you must be ready to deal with upper airway obstruction following extubation.

Effective Airway Clearance

Patients must have an effective cough if they are to clear secretions after the endotracheal tube is removed. Although this is difficult to assess while they are intubated, the answers to these three questions will help you predict how a patient will do after extubation:

- What is the patient's level of alertness?
- How strong is the patient's cough during suctioning?
- How often does the patient need to be suctioned?

For example, a patient who is wide awake, has a vigorous cough with suctioning, and has minimal airway secretions will almost certainly have no difficulty maintaining airway clearance following extubation. On the other hand, a patient who is very lethargic, requires frequent suctioning, and has little or no cough response, should not be extubated even if they do well on an SBT. Of course, there's a large gray area between these two extremes, but the answers to these questions will at least give you a framework for judging the advisability of extubation.

The Difficult Airway

A patient is said to have a "difficult airway" when they cannot be adequately ventilated with a bag-mask, intubated using standard laryngoscopy, or both. This can result from a number of factors, including morbid obesity, a recessed mandible (retrognathia), and temporo-mandibular joint or cervical spine immobility. Critical care physicians are trained to screen for these problems prior to intubation, but it's essential that this assessment also be performed before extubation. Information about prior intubation attempts is, of course, invaluable, so be sure to review the medical record and speak with your colleagues. This pre-extubation assessment is important because patients with a difficult airway have a high risk of morbidity and even death if re-intubation is required. So make sure that you have all the equipment and personnel needed before extubating a patient with a known or suspected difficult airway.

Sir William Osler once said, "Medicine is an art of probability," and this certainly pertains to the process of determining whether or not a patient should be extubated. Despite your best clinical judgment and lots of experience, some patients who are judged ready for extubation will subsequently need to be re-intubated. There are undoubtedly patients in whom the opposite is true. For your reference (and consolation), most studies report extubation failure rates of 5–15%. It's often said that if you are not re-intubating a few patients, you probably are not extubating soon enough!

Approach to the Difficult-to-Wean Patient

Unfortunately, many patients cannot be quickly removed from mechanical ventilation. This may be because the underlying reason for intubation has failed to improve or because the patient has developed one or more new problems while on the ventilator. Often, both occur. When faced with a patient who consistently does poorly during SBTs, your goal is to determine the reason(s) for ventilator-dependence and then come up with a therapeutic strategy.

To begin this process, it's very useful to think of ventilator-dependence as being the result of an abnormal relationship between ventilatory ability and ventilatory demand (Figure 15.2). *Ventilatory ability* is the minute ventilation ($\dot{V}_E$) that a patient can maintain for an indefinite period of time. *Ventilatory demand* is the $\dot{V}_E$ needed to excrete CO_2 and maintain an acceptable $PaCO_2$ and arterial pH. Normally, of course, ability far outstrips demand. That's why breathing is usually so effortless. Ventilator-dependence occurs when

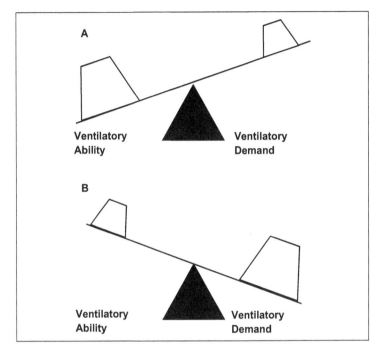

Figure 15.2 (A) Normally, ventilatory ability far exceeds ventilatory demand.
(B) Ventilator-dependence occurs when demand exceeds ability.

a patient's ventilatory demand exceeds their ability. This may be caused by increased demand, impaired ability, or (often) both.

Like routine weaning, the evaluation and management of the ventilator-dependent patient can be broken down into several steps (Figure 15.3).

Step 1: Assess Ventilatory Ability and Demand

Ventilatory demand is determined by noting the $\dot{V}_E$ needed during assisted mechanical ventilation to generate an "appropriate" $PaCO_2$. For most patients, of course, this is around 40 mmHg, but it may be either higher (e.g., in a patient with chronic hypercapnia) or lower (e.g., during compensation for a metabolic acidosis). If you keep in mind that $\dot{V}_E$ is normally in the range of 6–8 L/min, you can get a good sense of whether your patient's requirements are excessive. Next, measure $\dot{V}_E$ during totally unassisted breathing using a pressure support level of zero. Now compare these two numbers. In patients who have repeatedly failed attempts to discontinue mechanical ventilation, demand will almost always exceed ability, and it will be obvious why the patient cannot maintain spontaneous ventilation.

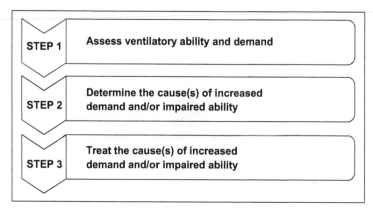

Figure 15.3 The three steps for evaluating and treating the difficult-to-wean patient.

Step 2: Determine the Cause(s) of Increased Demand, Impaired Ability, or Both

Table 15.3 lists the causes of impaired ventilatory ability and excessive demand. Carefully evaluate your patient. Can you explain their abnormal ability–demand relationship? In most cases, patients have several reasons for ventilator-dependence. I'll now discuss the most common causes.

Reduced Ability

Over-Sedation, Delirium, and Encephalopathy

These three conditions are extremely common in ICU patients and can have a profound effect on our ability to wean them from mechanical ventilation. Regardless of the cause, any process that impairs alertness is likely to reduce spontaneous tidal volume. Spontaneous respiratory rate may also fall, but it typically increases to compensate for the drop in tidal volume.

Critical Illness Polyneuropathy and Myopathy

Clinically significant muscle weakness due to critical illness polyneuropathy (CIP), critical illness myopathy (CIM), or both, is believed to occur in as many as one-third of mechanically ventilated patients. Since involvement of the diaphragm and the other respiratory muscles is common, these disorders are a very important cause of ventilator-dependence. Although their pathogenesis remains unclear, the most important risk factor for CIM is the use of corticosteroids and neuromuscular blocking agents, whereas CIP occurs primarily in patients with the systemic inflammatory response syndrome (SIRS) or severe sepsis.

Since isolated diaphragm weakness is rare, patients with persistent ventilator-dependence can be screened for CIP and CIM simply by assessing their peripheral muscle strength, and the diagnosis can usually be confirmed with electromyography and nerve-conduction studies. The treatment of CIM and

Table 15.3 Causes of Ventilator-Dependence

Category		Causes	Examples
Reduced Ability	Neuromuscular disease	Altered mental status	Over-sedation, delirium, encephalopathy
		Inadequate respiratory drive	Over-sedation, delirium, encephalopathy
		Impaired conduction to the respiratory muscles	Critical illness polyneuropathy
		Respiratory muscle weakness	Critical illness myopathy
	Lung disease	Obstructive lung disease	COPD, asthma, bronchiectasis
		Restrictive lung disease	Interstitial lung disease, organizing lung injury, interstitial edema
		Air space filling diseases	Pulmonary edema, pneumonia, atelectasis
	Chest wall disease	Morbid obesity	
		Large pleural effusions	
		Massive ascites	
	Cardiovascular disease	LV failure	Cardiomyopathy, ischemia, diastolic dysfunction
Increased Demand	Metabolic acidosis		Renal failure, dilutional acidosis, diarrhea
	Hyperventilation		Pain, anxiety, iatrogenic
	Elevated dead space ventilation	Significant underlying lung disease	
	Hyper-metabolic states		Fever, infection, hyperthyroidism

CIP is supportive and both conditions usually improve over a period of weeks to months.

Lung Disease

Ventilator-associated pneumonia and atelectasis are common in patients with respiratory failure and may cause or contribute to ventilator-dependence. Unfortunately, these disorders are often unrecognized because they may not be evident on a portable chest radiograph. Computed tomography, with its significantly greater sensitivity and specificity, can be very helpful in identifying or excluding these disorders. Also, make sure that you have optimized bronchodilator and anti-inflammatory therapy in patients with underlying obstructive lung disease.

Chest Wall Disease

Morbid obesity, pleural effusions, and ascites all reduce chest wall compliance, so during spontaneous breathing, much more inspiratory effort is needed to generate an acceptable tidal volume. Not surprisingly, this often leads to rapid, shallow breathing and repeated SBT failure. Draining large effusions and ascites can aid the weaning process. In morbidly obese patients, it is essential to perform SBTs in an upright position, either in the bed, or better yet, in a chair. This shifts weight off the chest wall, improves compliance, and increases tidal volume.

LV Dysfunction

Systolic and/or diastolic heart failure leading to pulmonary edema is another common, treatable, and often unrecognized cause of ventilator-dependence. Echocardiographic assessment of LV function is mandatory in all difficult-to-wean patients.

Increased Demand

Metabolic Acidosis

The respiratory system compensates for metabolic acidosis by increasing minute ventilation, which decreases the $PaCO_2$ and increases the arterial pH. Although it's well-tolerated in patients with normal lung function, this increase in required $\dot{V}_E$ may lead to ventilator-dependence in patients with limited ventilatory reserve. Renal failure, diarrhea, and large infusions of crystalloid ("dilutional acidosis") are the most common causes of persistent metabolic acidosis, and correcting the acidosis can be very helpful in some patients with ventilator-dependence.

Hyperventilation

Like respiratory compensation for metabolic acidosis, hyperventilation during mechanical ventilation causes the $PaCO_2$ to fall, increases the required $\dot{V}_E$, and may impair the weaning process. The mechanism is a little different, though. Chronic hyperventilation and the resulting respiratory alkalosis lead to decreased renal reabsorption of bicarbonate and a fall in the serum bicarbonate concentration. During an SBT, the patient must then maintain the preexisting low $PaCO_2$ in order to keep the arterial pH normal, and this increases ventilatory demand.

During mechanical ventilation, persistent hyperventilation may be caused by excessive patient-triggering in the setting of uncontrolled anxiety or pain. In such cases, providing adequate sedation or analgesia will usually correct the problem. Much more commonly, hyperventilation results from an inappropriately high set respiratory rate (iatrogenic hyperventilation). You should always suspect this when your patient's total and set respiratory rate are the same. When this happens, simply reduce the set rate until the patient begins to trigger additional, spontaneous breaths.

As discussed in Chapter 13, it's very important to remember that hyperventilation can cause not only a truly low $PaCO_2$ (i.e., <40 mmHg) but also a $PaCO_2$ that is less than normal *for the patient*. For example, a $PaCO_2$ of 50 mmHg would be abnormally low for a patient with severe COPD and a baseline $PaCO_2$ of 80 mmHg. If this low $PaCO_2$ persists, the serum bicarbonate concentration will fall, and during an SBT, the patient will have a ventilation requirement that they couldn't maintain even before they got sick and ended up on the ventilator. It should be obvious that such a patient has no chance of weaning from mechanical ventilation until both the $PaCO_2$ and the serum bicarbonate concentration are restored to their baseline levels. How do you identify this problem? The best way is to find blood gas measurements that were done prior to the patient's current hospitalization. If these aren't available, review previous serum bicarbonate concentrations and make sure that there hasn't been a significant change.

Increased Dead Space Ventilation
Recall from Chapter 2 that any disorder that affects the airways, parenchyma, or vasculature of the lungs causes both abnormally low and abnormally high ventilation-perfusion ($\dot{V}/\dot{Q}$) ratios. This leads to arterial hypoxemia, an increase in wasted or "dead space" ventilation, and an increase in the $\dot{V}_E$ needed to maintain a given $PaCO_2$. So, you can see that lung disease can not only reduce the sustainable $\dot{V}_E$, as discussed previously, it can also increase ventilatory demand. That's why it's so important to diagnose and effectively treat any type of lung disease when a patient is having difficulty coming off of mechanical ventilation.

Hyper-Metabolic States
Fever, uncontrolled infection, and hyperthyroidism increase total CO_2 production. This increases the $\dot{V}_E$ needed to maintain an appropriate $PaCO_2$. Ventilatory demand often falls significantly once these problems have been recognized and treated.

Step 3: Treat the Causes of Increased Demand and Impaired Ability

The evaluation described in Step 2 will often identify not just one, but several potential causes of increased ventilatory demand and impaired ability. Your job is to now do everything you can to correct these problems. If you are able to restore a more normal relationship between demand and ability, your patient has a good chance of resuming spontaneous ventilation, and the weaning process should be continued. If the problems you've identified cannot be treated, or if demand still exceeds ability following therapy, you can conclude that the patient is likely to remain ventilator-dependent and that additional weaning attempts are unlikely to be successful.

When to Perform a Tracheostomy

As outlined in Box 15.2, tracheostomy has many advantages over trans-laryngeal intubation with an endotracheal tube. On the other hand, tracheostomy is a surgical procedure and carries a small risk of complications, including bleeding, infection, pneumothorax, and tracheal stenosis. There is nearly universal agreement that patients who have difficulty weaning from mechanical ventilation should undergo tracheostomy. *When* it should be done continues to be

> ### Box 15.2 Advantages of Tracheostomy
>
> - Improved patient comfort
> - Reduced sedation needs
> - More effective patient communication
>   - "Lip reading" becomes easier
>   - Speech may be possible
> - Improved patient mobility
>   - Patients can safely get out bed and even ambulate
> - The patient may be able to eat and drink

the subject of debate and controversy. That's because the results of randomized, controlled trials of early (2–8 days) versus late (13–16 days) tracheostomy have been inconsistent and contradictory.

I favor an individualized approach. Patients who are alert, able to interact and communicate, and get out of bed are most likely to benefit from the advantages shown in Box 15.2. They should have a tracheostomy performed as soon as you are convinced that they will not be able to sustain spontaneous ventilation for at least a few weeks. Patients who are less alert and more debilitated will derive little benefit from early tracheostomy, and the procedure can be delayed, especially if the cause of respiratory failure is improving. When respiratory failure has been caused by a chronic disease (e.g., Guillain-Barre syndrome or spinal cord injury), there is no reason to delay the procedure, and regardless of patient characteristics, tracheostomy should be performed as soon as possible.

Additional Reading

Artime CA, Hagberg CA. Tracheal extubation. *Respir Care*. 2014;59:991–1005.

McConville JF, Kress JP. Weaning patients from the ventilator. *N Engl J Med*. 2012;367:2233–2239.

Perren A, Brochard L. Managing the apparent and hidden difficulties of weaning from mechanical ventilation. *Intensive Care Med*. 2013;39:1885–1895.

Chapter 16

Noninvasive Mechanical Ventilation

Up until now, every chapter of this book has focused on mechanical ventilation delivered through an endotracheal tube. Although so-called invasive ventilation can be life-saving, it can also cause significant morbidity. For example, bypassing the upper airway greatly increases the risk of ventilator-associated pneumonia. Furthermore, the sedation that is almost invariably required prolongs the duration of mechanical ventilation, increases the risk of delirium and long-term cognitive impairment, and contributes to the generalized weakness and debilitation that are so common following critical illness.

It has long been recognized that positive-pressure ventilation can also be delivered "non-invasively" to critically ill patients through several different types of "interfaces" (usually a tight-fitting face mask). In theory, at least, this should reduce the need for intubation and decrease the risks associated with invasive mechanical ventilation.

During the past 30 years, studies have shown that noninvasive ventilation (NIV) is beneficial when used to treat selected patients with respiratory failure, and its use has become increasingly common. Today, NIV is an essential part of ICU care, but it's also used in many other venues, including the prehospital setting, emergency department, post-operative care unit, and medical and surgical wards.

This chapter describes the machines and circuits used to deliver NIV, reviews its indications and contraindications, and explains how to initiate and adjust NIV.

Noninvasive Mechanical Ventilators

Bi-level Ventilators

Noninvasive ventilation is a lot more complicated than simply substituting a face mask for an endotracheal tube. In fact, until fairly recently, ICU ventilators were unable to deliver NIV. That's why specialized ventilators were developed specifically for this purpose. These machines are usually referred to as "bi-level" ventilators, because, as shown in Figure 16.1, they generate two different, clinician-set levels of airway pressure (P_{AW}).

Most bi-level ventilators have their own set of terms and abbreviations. The pressure during inspiration is usually referred to as the *inspiratory positive airway pressure*, or IPAP, and the pressure throughout expiration is the

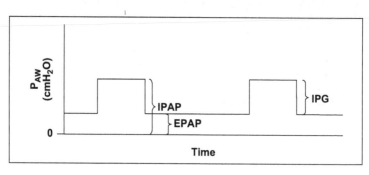

Figure 16.1 Plot of airway pressure (P$_{AW}$) versus time produced by a noninvasive, bi-level ventilator.

IPAP = inspiratory positive airway pressure; EPAP = expiratory positive airway pressure; IPG = inspiratory pressure gradient

expiratory positive airway pressure, or EPAP. As you can see from Figure 16.1, EPAP is simply another name for PEEP. The difference between IPAP and EPAP is the *inspiratory pressure gradient,* which drives gas into the lungs during each mechanical breath. Bi-level ventilators should not be confused with CPAP (continuous positive airway pressure) machines, which maintain a constant pressure level throughout the entire respiratory cycle. Since there is no gradient between inspiration and expiration, CPAP machines provide no inspiratory assistance.

There are several important differences between bi-level and conventional ICU ventilators. We'll start with the ventilator circuit (Figure 16.2). Remember from Chapter 4 that ICU ventilators have a circuit with separate inspiratory and expiratory limbs and an integrated expiratory valve. Bi-level ventilators use a single-limb circuit, which, instead of an expiratory valve, has an *exhalation port* that is adjacent to the mask. The exhalation port is always open, so there is a constant gas leak from the circuit. In NIV jargon, this is referred to as an "intentional" leak to distinguish it from the "unintentional" leaks that usually occur around the mask.

ICU ventilators provide gas flow only during inspiration while the expiratory valve is closed. Since the circuit is closed, all the gas from the ventilator enters the patient's lungs. When inspiration ends, flow stops, the expiratory valve opens to allow exhalation, and then closes again to maintain a clinician-set level of PEEP. In contrast, bi-level machines provide gas flow throughout both inspiration and expiration. Since the circuit is open (i.e., it has a continuous intentional gas leak), the pressure in the ventilator circuit is determined by the *net flow*—that is, the difference between the total flow provided by the ventilator and the flow passing through the exhalation port. During inspiration, flow increases to achieve the set inspiratory pressure. When inspiration ends, flow falls until the set expiratory pressure is reached. Tidal volume is

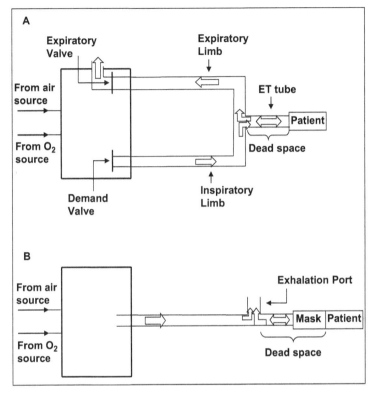

Figure 16.2 (A) ICU ventilators use a double-limb circuit with a demand valve and an expiratory valve. Equipment dead space equals the volume of the endotracheal (ET) tube and any tubing between the patient and the junction of the inspiratory and expiratory limbs.

(B) Bi-level ventilators use a single-limb circuit. Gas flows from the ventilator throughout the respiratory cycle, and a portion exits through the exhalation port. Exhaled gas also leaves through the exhalation port. Equipment dead space equals the volume of the mask and the circuit between the patient and the exhalation port. In both figures, the arrows show the direction and magnitude of gas flow.

directly proportional to the pressure (and flow) gradient between inspiration and expiration.

The circuits used by ICU and bi-level ventilators also differ in the amount of dead space they create. You can think of this as the volume of exhaled gas that's inhaled or "rebreathed" at the beginning of each breath. Since endotracheal and tracheostomy tubes contain less volume than the normal upper airway, dead space is actually reduced with invasive ventilation. During NIV, though, *potential* dead space is increased because exhaled gas enters the mask and the ventilator circuit proximal to the exhalation port (Figure 16.2B). This would ordinarily cause the patient to rebreathe exhaled CO_2, reduce the efficiency of CO_2 excretion, and increase the minute ventilation needed to maintain a normal arterial PCO_2. This doesn't happen, though, because of the constant gas flow that's maintained throughout expiration. This flow not only generates EPAP, it also washes exhaled gas from the mask and circuit and prevents CO_2 rebreathing. On most machines, an EPAP of at least 4 cmH_2O is recommended to ensure adequate CO_2 wash-out.

The most important distinguishing feature of bi-level ventilators is that they are "leak-tolerant." The magnitude of both the intentional and unintentional leaks depends on many factors, including the set airway pressure, the duration of inspiration, the type of mask, and patient characteristics that can prevent a tight fit, such as a beard, or the absence of teeth or dentures. Furthermore, the volume lost from the system often varies from breath to breath. Bi-level ventilators compensate for this variable leakage by continuously monitoring inspiratory and expiratory flow, inspired and expired volume, and circuit pressure both within the machine and at the exhalation port. Proprietary algorithms then rapidly adjust flow to maintain the set levels of inspiratory and expiratory pressure.

Modes and Breath Types

Modern bi-level ventilators allow the clinician to select from several different modes and breath types. As with conventional ICU ventilators, terminology varies among manufacturers. Most bi-level machines used in the ICU provide the following options (as defined in Chapter 5):

- CMV-PC—Patients receive a clinician-set number of mandatory pressure control breaths but may trigger any number of additional pressure control breaths (Figure 16.3A).
- SIMV-PC—Patients receive a clinician-set number of mandatory pressure control breaths but may trigger any number of additional pressure support breaths (Figure 16.3B).

ICU Ventilators and Noninvasive Ventilation

I told you before that noninvasive ventilation is more complicated than just substituting a mask for an endotracheal tube. In fact, if we were to do that with a standard ICU ventilator and double-limb circuit, the unintentional gas leak around the mask could cause significant problems during every phase of the respiratory cycle.

- Triggering—ICU ventilators provide a mechanical breath when inspiratory effort lowers either P_{AW} or the base flow below a clinician-set level. By allowing room air to enter the mask during inspiration, a large leak would reduce the drop in P_{AW} or flow produced by patient effort. This

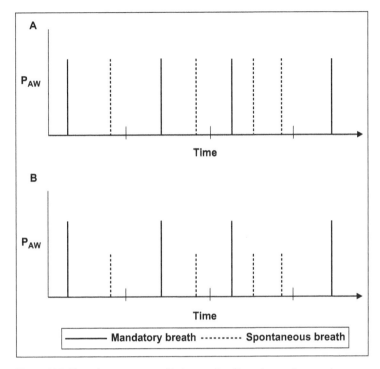

Figure 16.3 Plots of airway pressure (P_{AW}) versus time illustrating mandatory and spontaneous breaths during (A) CMV-PC and (B) SIMV-PC.

would effectively reduce ventilator sensitivity and lead to ineffective triggering and increased patient work of breathing. On the other hand, a leak during expiration could cause breaths to be "auto-triggered" by lowering P_{AW} or the base flow.

- Inspiration—The volume entering the patient's lungs would be reduced by the volume that leaks around the mask.
- Transition from inspiration to expiration—Since pressure support breaths are flow-cycled, inspiration ends and expiration begins only when flow falls below a minimum, set level. When a leak is present, there will always be a pressure gradient driving flow between the ventilator, the mask, and the outside air, and this could prevent flow from reaching the level needed to cycle a conventional ICU ventilator.

• Expiration—ICU ventilators maintain a set level of PEEP by closing the expiratory valve before the respiratory system returns to its resting or equilibrium volume. If there's a leak around the mask, gas will flow out of the lungs even after the expiratory valve closes, and PEEP will progressively fall toward zero (atmospheric pressure).

Within the past few years, manufacturers of ICU ventilators have added software with algorithms that have made these machines much more leak-tolerant. Consequently, the inherent problems with triggering, cycling, inadequate volume delivery, and maintenance of PEEP have been largely eliminated, and these ventilators can now be used for both invasive and noninvasive ventilation. Since ICU ventilators use a circuit with separate inspiratory and expiratory limbs and an active exhalation valve, there is no need for an exhalation port with its intentional gas leak.

Modes and Breath Types

ICU ventilators vary with respect to the modes and breath types available during NIV, so it's important to know the options on your machine. In general, ventilators provide some or all of the mode-breath type combinations previously listed for bi-level machines. Some machines also allow:

• CMV-VC—Patients receive a clinician-set number of mandatory volume control breaths but may trigger any number of additional volume control breaths.
• SIMV-VC—Patients receive a clinician-set number of mandatory volume control breaths but may trigger any number of additional pressure support breaths.

Patient Selection

Box 16.1 lists the general indications for NIV. Noninvasive ventilation is predominantly used to treat or prevent hypercapnia and respiratory acidosis in patients with established or impending ventilation or oxygenation-ventilation failure. It is used less often to improve arterial PO_2 and SaO_2 in patients with oxygenation failure. Generally accepted contraindications to NIV are listed in Box 16.2.

Box 16.1 General Indications for NIV

• Acute or acute-on-chronic hypercapnia and respiratory acidosis
• Impending hypercapnia and respiratory acidosis
  • Marked dyspnea and tachypnea
  • Increased work of breathing
• Oxygenation failure

Box 16.2 Contraindications to NIV

Absolute

- Cardiac or respiratory arrest (established or impending)
- Facial surgery, trauma, or deformity
- Upper airway obstruction
- Vomiting or high risk of vomiting

Relative

- Hypotension
- Inability to cooperate
- Ineffective cough and airway clearance
- Depressed level of consciousness

Summary of Available Evidence

When compared with standard medical therapy, randomized controlled trials have shown that NIV decreases the need for intubation and reduces mortality in patients with:

- Hypercapnic acidosis caused by an exacerbation of COPD
- Cardiogenic pulmonary edema

The effectiveness of NIV in patients with established or impending hypercapnic acidosis from other causes, such as asthma, neuromuscular diseases, restrictive chest wall diseases, and obesity-hypoventilation syndrome, is less clear. That's because, depending on the disease, there are either insufficient data or studies have reported conflicting results. Despite this lack of evidence, it's clear that, for many patients with these disorders, NIV can improve dyspnea, tachypnea, and gas exchange and may eliminate the need for intubation. In the absence of contraindications, a trial of NIV is warranted in most patients.

The role of NIV in patients with oxygenation failure is more controversial. Some randomized controlled trials and observational studies have shown improved outcomes and reduced need for intubation in patients with pneumonia and even mild ARDS, whereas others have failed to demonstrate these benefits. What's concerning, though, is that failure to improve with NIV is associated with significantly increased mortality. This has suggested to some investigators that NIV causes an unsafe delay in intubating patients with progressive, hypoxemic respiratory failure. If NIV does, in fact, reduce the need for intubation in some patients, it's likely that this benefit occurs within a relatively narrow window during the course of the disease. Since this "sweet spot" has not been identified, NIV should be used with caution in this patient population. A brief, closely monitored trial may be worthwhile, but lack of significant, objective improvement requires immediate intubation and invasive mechanical ventilation.

How to Initiate, Monitor, and Adjust Noninvasive Ventilation

The Patient–Ventilator Interface

Either a *full* (covers nose and mouth) or a *total* (covers nose, mouth, and eyes) face mask should be used. It's important to select the type and size that optimize patient comfort while minimizing gas leaks.

Ventilator Settings

Bi-level Ventilators

In patients with established or impending hypercapnic acidosis, the ventilator should ideally be set to provide an adequate number of guaranteed breaths, each with a tidal volume of 400–500 ml. This can be done using any of the mode–breath type combinations that were previously described. Suggested initial settings are shown in Table 16.1. Note that you must set the IPAP and EPAP and that the tidal volume is proportional to the difference between these pressures (the inspiratory pressure gradient). On SIMV-PC, the pressure support level must also be specified. It's important to assess the effect of these initial settings within 10–15 minutes and make changes, as needed.

If the patient requires additional *ventilation* because of persistent or worsening dyspnea, tachypnea, or respiratory acidosis, increase the IPAP in increments of 3–5 cmH_2O. Tidal volume and minute ventilation will usually increase in proportion to the inspiratory pressure gradient. IPAP should be increased as often as every 10 minutes and titrated to clinical effect.

If *oxygenation* is inadequate, incrementally increase the EPAP by 3–5 cmH_2O. This will augment alveolar recruitment, reduce shunt fraction, and improve the PaO_2 and SaO_2. It's important to remember that when EPAP is changed, most bi-level ventilators do not automatically adjust the IPAP to keep the inspiratory pressure gradient constant. This means that you must always change the EPAP and IPAP by the same amount if you want to maintain the same level of inspiratory support.

Table 16.1 Initial Settings on a Bi-Level Ventilator		
Mode	**CMV-PC**	**SIMV-PC**
Mandatory rate (bpm)	14	14
F_iO_2	1.0	1.0
IPAP (cmH_2O)	12	12
EPAP (cmH_2O)	5	5
PS level (cmH_2O)		12

IPAP = inspiratory positive airway pressure; EPAP = expiratory positive airway pressure; PS = pressure support

Table 16.2 Initial Settings on ICU Ventilators (NIV-capable)

Mode	CMV-PC	SIMV-PC
Mandatory rate (bpm)	14	14
F_iO_2	1.0	1.0
Driving pressure (cmH$_2$O)	7	7
PEEP (cmH$_2$O)	5	5
PS level (cmH$_2$O)		12

PEEP = positive end-expiratory pressure; PS = pressure support

In general, keep inspiratory airway pressure below 25–30 cmH$_2$O. Higher pressures are usually poorly tolerated, often produce an unacceptably high leak, and may lead to gastric inflation.

ICU Ventilators

If an ICU ventilator is used, you must first make sure that it's capable of and set to deliver NIV. Initial settings and subsequent adjustments are the same as when using bi-level ventilators. Unfortunately, the terminology usually differs, so it's important to become familiar with the options provided by your machine. Initial recommended settings are listed in Table 16.2.

Instead of setting total inspiratory pressure (IPAP), most ICU ventilators require that you specify the inspiratory pressure gradient. This is the driving pressure of pressure control breaths and the pressure support level of pressure support breaths. You must also set a PEEP level. Total inspiratory pressure is then the sum of the set inspiratory pressure gradient and PEEP. This allows you to adjust inspiratory support simply by changing the driving pressure or pressure support level, and changes in PEEP do not affect the inspiratory pressure gradient.

Monitoring

When used to treat acute or acute-on-chronic respiratory failure, NIV should always be initiated in the ICU. Patients must be closely monitored to assess their response to NIV and to determine appropriate adjustments in ventilator settings. Cardiac monitoring, continuous pulse oximetry, and airway-suction devices are essential, and equipment and personnel must be immediately available for endotracheal intubation, should the need arise. In patients with hypercapnic acidosis, arterial blood gases should be monitored closely for the first few hours to follow PaCO$_2$ and arterial pH, and an indwelling arterial catheter is usually needed.

Converting to Invasive Mechanical Ventilation

Although this decision must be made on a case-by-case basis, there are two important guiding principles. First, most patients should be intubated if they fail to improve or worsen during the first few hours of NIV, or if they develop additional contraindications to its use (e.g., depressed mental status or agitation, excessive secretions, hypotension). Second, always err on the side of performing early, elective intubation rather than waiting until rapid deterioration leads to a potentially life-threatening airway emergency.

Additional Reading

Cabrini L, Giovanni L, Oriani A, et al. Noninvasive ventilation and survival in acute care settings: A comprehensive systematic review and meta-analysis of randomized controlled trials. *Crit Care Med*. 2015;43:880–888.

Gregoretti C, Pisani L, Cortegiani A, Ranieri VM. Noninvasive ventilation in critically ill patients. *Crit Care Clin*. 2015;31:435–457.

Hess DR. Noninvasive ventilation for acute respiratory failure. *Respir Care*. 2013;58: 950–969.

Scala R, Naldi M. Ventilators for noninvasive ventilation to treat acute respiratory failure. *Respir Care*. 2008;53:1054–1080.

Index

Figures, tables, and boxes are indicated by an italic *f*, *t*, or *b* following the page number.